Springer
Milan
Berlin
Heidelberg
New York
Barcelona
Budapest
Hong Kong
London
Paris
Singapore
Tokyo

Atlas of Enteroscopy

Editors

F.P. Rossini • G. Gay

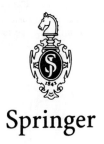

Springer

FRANCESCO P. ROSSINI, M.D.
Gastroenterology
Gastrointestinal Endoscopy Service
Department of Oncology
S. Giovanni A.S. Hospital
Via Cavour 31
10123 Turin
Italy

GERARD J. GAY, M.D.
Service de Médicine Interne L.
Hôpital Villemin
47, rue de Nabecor
54035 Nancy Cedex
France

ISBN 978-88-470-2193-8   ISBN 978-88-470-2191-4 (eBook)
DOI 10.1007/978-88-470-2191-4

© Springer-Verlag Italia, Milano 1998
Softcover reprint of the hardcover 1st edition 1998

Library of Congress Cataloging-in-Publication Data: Atlas of enteroscopy / F.P. Rossini , G. Gay (eds.). p. cm. Includes bibliographical references and index.   1. Enteroscopy--Atlases. 2. Intestine, Small--Diseases--Diagnosis--Atlases.
I. Rossini, Francesco Paolo. II. Gay, G. (Gerard), 1945-[DNLM: 1. Gastrointestinal Diseases--diagnosis atlases. 2. Malabsorption Syndromes--diagnosis atlases. 3. Endoscopy, Gastrointestinal atlases. 4. Intestine, Small--radiography atlases. WI 17 A8785 1998] RC804.
E64A87 1988 616.3'30754-dc21 DNLM/DLC for Library of Congress 98-20746 CIP

This work is subject to copyright. All rights are reserved, whether the whole or part of the material is concerned, specifically the rights of translation, reprinting, re-use of illustrations, recitation, broadcasting, reproduction on microfilms or in other ways, and storage in data banks. Duplication of this publication or parts thereof is only permitted under the provisions of the Italian Copyright Law in its current version, and permission for use must always be obtained from Springer-Verlag. Violations are liable for prosecution under the Italian Copyright Law.

The use of general descriptive names, registered names, trademarks, etc. in this publication does not imply, even in the absence of a specific statement, that such names are exempt from the relevant protective laws and regulations and therefore free for general use.

Product liability: The publisher cannot guarantee the accuracy of any information about dosage and application contained in this book. In every individual case the user must check such information by consulting the relevant literature.

Typesetting: Photo Life (Milan)

Cover design: Simona Colombo

SPIN: 10662854

Preface

The aim of this book is to provide a brief and clear message and an updated view of the diagnostic possibilities of enteroscopy: the last, or perhaps latest frontier of digestive endoscopy.

Until the 1990s, the recent past was characterized by numerous attempts to achieve an endoscopic view of the small bowel until technological innovations made it accessible via push and sonde enteroscopy.

The fact that we are now able to insert an enteroscope into the small bowel undoubtedly both increases the diagnostic possibilities and lays a solid foundation for research, in particular through histopathobiology.

By defining patterns indicative of various diseases, enteroscopy contributes to achieving a positive, constructive interdisciplinary collaboration between gastroenterology and other medical disciplines.

By systematically flanking endoscopic, radiological, echographic and morphological findings, all with close clinical connections, and with the support of reliably documented results, the aim of the *Atlas of Enteroscopy* is to stress the clinical role of enteroscopy through images.

The authors express their sincere thanks to all European experts in gastroenterology and enteroscopy whose excellent contributions have made it possible to realize this book, providing a splendid documentation that derives from solid experience in studying small bowel disease.

Our warm thanks also go to Olympus for giving us very considerable technological support and for their constant and active collaboration.

The work of Springer-Verlag Italia has been admirable in its professionalism, and as a result this *Atlas* is in the finest graphic tradition of this publishing house.

Francesco P. Rossini
Chief, Gastroenterology - Gastrointestinal Service
S. Giovanni A.S. Hospital, Turin
Professor of Gastroenterology, Post-Graduated School of
Internal Medicine, University of Turin
President, European Club of Enteroscopy

Gerard J. Gay
Chief, Dept. of Internal Medicine,
Centre Hospitalier Regional et Universitaire, Nancy, France
Professor of Therapeutics, University of Nancy
Secretary, European Club of Enteroscopy

Foreword

This book is a tribute to the extraordinary dedication of Professors Rossini and Gay to enteroscopy. They have done much to develop and advance this field of endoscopy. Doctors Rossini and Gay realized the potential of enteroscopy long ago and have been at the forefront of the worldwide acceptance of this methodology through their writings, teaching and their deep involvement in the procedure. The editors have drawn together a remarkable number of European authors who are renowned for their work in diseases of the small bowel, both diagnostic and therapeutic. Their vast collective experience provides an encompassing view of all the afflictions that can affect the small intestine. The information ranges from small bowel tumors to malabsorption and includes chapters on small bowel transplantation, AIDS, and other diagnostic methodologies. The lavish use of endophotographs shows intralumenal sights never published previously. A book of this breadth would have not have been possible a few years ago.

The indications for the three major types of enteroscopy have recently been collated and reformulated. The reasons for performing push enteroscopy, sonde enteroscopy, and intraoperative enteroscopy are on a more solid and scientific basis than ever before. The most current approaches to small bowel disorders are detailed both in the text and in the informative algorithms. Each facet of enteroscopy is extensively explored, as are the diseases that may be encountered during the examination. This volume is a repository for knowledge about enteroscopy and contains such a depth of information that anyone who treats patients will be able to learn something about the subject, whether they be fellows in gastroenterology, surgeons, or skilled enteroscopists. The subject of push enteroscopy is an example of the multiple layers of complexity the editors have built into the book: the major indications and usefulness of push enteroscopy are in the evaluation of obscure gastrointestinal bleeding; however, various chapters explore a myriad of other uses for this procedure and detail both the endoscopic and bioptic findings that can be encountered in other puzzling diagnostic problems.

The impact of the cumulative experience of the authors and the richness of the illustrations make this volume a landmark in the field of enteroscopy. We who have been involved as pioneers and developers of enteroscopy appreciate the depth of this book and the insight of the two editors. Together they have presented, in both written and pictorial form, the vast amount of knowledge that has been accumulated through the use of enteroscopy. Those who see and treat patients with obscure GI bleeding and diseases of the small bowel will find these pages filled with up-to-date information on these issues. The real beneficiaries of the knowledge contained within these pages will be patients with diseases of the small intestine whose diagnoses will be made and therapy instituted by those physicians and surgeons who have read and learned from this book.

Jerome D. Waye, M. D.
Clinical Professor of Medicine, The Mount Sinai Medical Center
Chief, Endoscopy Unit, Mount Sinai Hospital
Chief, Endoscopy Unit, Lenox Hill Hospital
Past President, American Society for Gastrointestinal Endoscopy
Past President, American College of Gastroenterology

In the history of medicine, the small intestine has always been a difficult organ to study. For many centuries, a diagnosis of diseases involving the small intestine was based on an anamnestic study of the subjective and objective symptoms. This information was then compared with that provided, as time passed, first by autopsy, then by radiology and surgical findings, and finally (!) by "in vivo" biopsies, which could often only be performed with relatively complex and contrived techniques.

For about ten years now, thanks to enteroscopy, we have finally had a means of "seeing" what normal and pathological intestinal mucosa looks like, "in vivo" and "in real time" and, above all, of carrying out "targeted" biopsies of the main lesions. Essentially, what has already occurred with the organs of the digestive tract that are more accessible to the endoscope, i.e., the esophagus, stomach, duodenum, rectum-colon and even the last portion of the ileum, is now also occurring for the small intestine. I say "is occurring" and not "has occurred" because enteroscopy is not as simple a technique as endoscopy: it requires more manual skill and takes much longer to carry out, patient compliance is lower and the equipment is very expensive both to buy and to maintain.

Nevertheless, ever since the first enteroscopic findings began to appear and macroscopic and microscopic data on the targeted biopsy specimens have finally become available, a great deal of new information has undoubtedly emerged. This has been the case in extensive diseases, for which a diagnosis was formerly based mainly on the findings that emerged from studying the first and last portions of the digestive tract, i.e., the duodenum and terminal ileum, but also in segmetary diseases, such as polyps and malignant and endocrine tumors, angiodysplasias and bleeding, complications and involutions of extensive diseases.

When I said "is occurring", I was referring to the increase in application that "is occurring" with enteroscopy. However, like all other diagnostic procedures, more precise and systematic information on the method and on the results achieved was necessary. What was missing was a reference book, simple and relatively concise but at the same time complete and with the characteristics of an atlas, i.e., with plenty of convincing illustrations since we are dealing with a morphological study. This had to provide the new information, integrate it with the traditional knowledge of the diseases of the small intestine, and compare it with the other morphological studies that we have been using for many years and also the newer radiological procedures, such as CT or MRI, etc.

This atlas volume is now presented to the medical world, by some of the most prestigious experts who have been dedicated to this sector for many years now. It is intended for anyone who wants to know more about this procedure – from the general practitioner to the most sophisticated clinical specialist.

"When something is well done, is simple, attractive and well presented, it is of use to everyone". This is an old saying that has, once again, proven to be right!

Giovanni Gasbarrini
Clinical Professor of Medicine, Catholic University, Rome
Head of the School of Internal Medicine and
Gastroenterology, Catholic University, Rome
President of the "Club del tenue"
Vice-President of the Gastro-Surgical Club

Contents

THE NORMAL SMALL BOWEL

The small bowel: structure and function (*F. Bonvicini, M. Baraldini*) 3

DIAGNOSTIC METHODOLOGIES

Small bowel imaging procedures (*D. Regent*) 17

Transabdominal ultrasonography (*V. Arienti*) 25

Nuclear tests (*G. Sciarretta, A. Furno*) 31

ENTEROSCOPY

Sonde enteroscopy (*J.F. MacKenzie*) 37

Push enteroscopy (*G. Gay, M. Pennazio, J.S. Delmotte, F.P. Rossini*) 43

Intraoperative enteroscopy (*G. Gay, M. Pennazio, J.S. Delmotte, F.P. Rossini*) 51

Laparoscopically assisted enteroscopy (*P. Bauret, J.M. Fabre*) 55

GASTROINTESTINAL BLEEDING

Emergency bleeding (*G. Gay, F.P. Rossini, J.S. Delmotte, M. Pennazio*) 61

Management of obscure gastrointestinal bleeding (*M. Pennazio, F.P. Rossini*) 63

Angiodysplasias (*A. Van Gossum, A. Schmit*) 69

NSAID enteropathy (*A.J. Morris*) 75

Meckel's diverticulum – Jejunoileal diverticulosis (*A. Arrigoni, F.P. Rossini*) 79

DIARRHEA AND MALABSORPTION

Diarrhea and malabsorption syndromes: clinical overview (*P. Mainguet*) 85

Diarrhea and malabsorption: the role of enteroscopy (*M. Pennazio, F.P. Rossini*) 89

Coeliac disease (*G.R. Corazza, M. Di Stefano, M.A. Pistoia*) 93

Tropical sprue (*F. Klotz*) 97

Whipple's disease (*G.R. Corazza, M. Di Stefano, M.A. Pistoia*) 99

Ulcerative jeunoileitis (*G.R. Corazza, M. Di Stefano, M.A. Pistoia*) 101

Eosinophilic enteropathy (*E. Brocchi, R. Corinaldesi*) 103

Vasculitis (*G. Gay, J.S. Delmotte*) 105

Crohn's disease (*A. Arrigoni, M. Pennazio, F.P. Rossini*) 107

Amyloidosis (*G. Gay, J.S. Delmotte*) 113

Sarcoidosis (*G. Gay, J.S. Delmotte*) 115

Mastocytosis (*G. Gay, J.S. Delmotte*) 117

Abeta and hypobetalipoproteinemias (*G. Gay, J.S. Delmotte*) 119

Hypogammaglobulinemia (*G. Gay, J.S. Delmotte*) 121

TUMORS

Small bowel tumors (*F.P. Rossini, M. Risio*) 125

Primary gastrointestinal lymphoma (*G. Gay, J.S. Delmotte*) 137

Carcinoid tumours of the small bowel (*G. Delle Fave, S. Angeletti*) 141

OTHER INDICATIONS

Enteroscopy and AIDS (*Ch. Florent*) 147

Enteroscopy of the transplanted small bowel
(*C.L. Scotti-Foglieni, S.D. Tinozzi, K. Abu-Elmagd, T.E. Starzl*) 151

Uncommon endoscopic appearances of the small bowel mucosa (*M. Pennazio, F.P. Rossini*) 171

Contributors

K. Abu-Elmagd
Thomas E. Starzl Transplantation Institute,
University of Pittsburgh School of Medicine,
Pittsburgh, Pennsylvania 15213, USA

S. Angeletti
Department of Gastroenterology, II Clinica Medica,
University "La Sapienza", Rome, Italy

V. Arienti
Centre of Research and Study in Abdominal
Ultrasonography, Department of Internal Medicine,
Cardioangiology, Hepatology, University of Bologna,
Bologna, Italy

A. Arrigoni
Gastroenterology-Gastrointestinal Endoscopy Service,
Department of Oncology, S. Giovanni A.S. Hospital,
Turin, Italy

M. Baraldini
Institute of Chemical Sciences, University of Bologna,
Bologna, Italy

P. Bauret
Fédération médico-chirurgicale des Maladies de l'Appareil Digestif, Hôpital Saint Eloi, Montpellier, France

F. Bonvicini
Department of Internal Medicine, Cardioangiology,
Hepatology, University of Bologna, Bologna, Italy

E. Brocchi
Department of Internal Medicine and Gastroenterology,
University of Bologna, Policlinico S. Orsola, Bologna,
Italy

G.R. Corazza
Department of Internal Medicine, University of L'Aquila,
L'Aquila, Italy

R. Corinaldesi
Patologia Medica II, Università degli Studi di Bologna,
Policlinico S. Orsola, Bologna, Italy

G. Delle Fave
Department of Gastroenterology, Department of Internal
Medicine 2, University "La Sapienza", Rome, Italy

J.-S. Delmotte
Endoscopy Unit, Clinique des Maladies de l'Appareil
Digestif, Hôpital Claude Huriet, CHRU de Lille,
Lille, France

M. Di Stefano
Department of Internal Medicine, University of L'Aquila,
L'Aquila, Italy

J.M. Fabre
Fédération médico-chirurgicale des Maladies de l'Appareil Digestif, Hôpital Saint Eloi, Montpellier, France

Ch. Florent
Saint Antoine Hospital, Service d'Hepato-Gastro-
entérologie, Paris, France

A. Furno
Nuclear Medicine Unit, Maggiore Hospital, Bologna, Italy

G. Gay
Service de Medicine Interne "L", Hôpital Villemin,
Nancy, France

F. Klotz
Medical Services, Hôpital Tropical Medicine Principal,
Dakar, Sénégal

P. Mainguet
Service de Gastro-entérologie, Cliniques Universitaires
Saint-Luc, Brussels, Belgium

A.J. Morris
Department of Gastroenterology, Royal Infirmary,
Glasgow, Scotland

J.F. MacKenzie
Department of Gastroenterology, Royal Infirmary,
Glasgow, Scotland

Contributors

M. Pennazio
Gastroenterology-Gastrointestinal Endoscopy Service, Department of Oncology, S. Giovanni A.S. Hospital, Turin, Italy

M.A. Pistoia
Department of Surgery, University of L'Aquila, L'Aquila, Italy

D. Regent
Service de Radiologie Adultes, Hôpital de Brabois, Vandoeuvre Cedex, France

M. Risio
Surgical Pathology Service, Department of encology, S. Giovanni A.S. Hospital, Turin, Italy

F.P. Rossini
Gastroenterology-Gastrointestinal Endoscopy Service, Department of Oncology, S. Giovanni A.S. Hospital, Turin, Italy

A. Schmit
Department of Gastroenterology and Hepatopancreatology, Erasme Hospital, Free University of Brussels, Brussels, Belgium

G. Sciarretta
Gastroenterology Unit, Maggiore Hospital, Bologna, Italy

C.L. Scotti-Foglieni
Institute of General Surgery and Organ Transplantation
University of Pavia School of Medicine and Surgery
Director, Transplantation Department, IRCCS Ospedale Policlinico "San Matteo" di Pavia
27100 Pavia, Italy

T.E. Starzl
Director
Thomas E. Starzl Transplantation Institute
University of Pittsburgh School of Medicine
Pittsburgh, Pennsylvania 15213, USA

S.D. Tinozzi
Institute of General Surgery and Organ Transplantation
University of Pavia School of Medicine and Surgery
Director, Division of Surgical Pathology, IRCCS Ospedale Policlinico "San Matteo" di Pavia
27100 Pavia, Italy

A. Van Gossum
Department of Gastroenterology and Hepatopancreatology, Erasme Hospital, Free University of Brussels, Brussels, Belgium

The Normal Small Bowel

The small bowel: structure and function

F. Bonvicini, M. Baraldini

Introduction

The structure of the small intestine clearly expresses the main function of this organ: absorption of nutrients introduced with the diet. The absorptive surface is extremely large due to the length of the tube, the amplification of the surface by *conniventes valvulae*, a further amplification by *villi*, and another amplification by *microvilli*.

On the other hand absorption is not the only function of the small bowel. Other functions are:
1. digestion: enterocyte plasma membrane enzymes, complete protein and carbohydrate digestion;
2. secretion: two types of exocrine secretions are present: water and electrolytes from crypts, mucus by goblet cells;
3. endocrine function: this is attested by the numerous cells of the digestive endocrine system which secrete peptide hormones or biogenic amines;
4. immune function: intraepithelial lymphocytes, plasma cells in lamina propria, lymphoepithelial organs disseminated along the tube and grouped in Peyer's patches in the distal small intestine attest this important function.

Anatomy

The small intestine begins after the pyloric sphincter and ends at the ileocecal valve. Its length ranges between 2 and 6 m. By convention the organ is subdivided into three segments: duodenum, jejunum and ileum. These segments lack a strong anatomical and structural demarcation, but this subdivision mainly expresses some anatomical and microscopic differences in structure and function. The passage from the duodenum to jejunum occurs at the so-called ligament of Treitz where the small intestine (duodenum) enters the peritoneal cavity. The ileum has a thinner wall with respect to the upper intestine; in fact, the distal duodenum and proximal jejunum contain the valves of Kerkring, which are constituted of mucosal circular folds. The jejunum has a wider lumen with respect to the ileum. On the other hand, the ileum is rich in lymphoepithelial organs (Peyer's patches).

As concerns **vascularization**, the duodenum is supplied by the celiac and superior mesenteric arteries. The jejunum is supplied by the superior mesenteric arteries from which the jejunal and ileal arteries originate, form arcades and give origin to *vasa recta* which penetrate into the intestinal wall. The terminal ileum is supplied by the ileocolic artery, arising from the lower portion of superior mesenteric artery.

The venous drainage from the small intestine occurs through the superior mesenteric vein, which joins the splenic vein and forms the portal vein. The lymphatics drain through lymph nodes to the thoracic duct.

As concerns the **nervous system**, the small intestine is innervated by extrinsic nerves, sympathetic and parasympathetic, of the autonomic system. The peculiar and most important innervation of small intestine is constituted by the intrinsic neurons of the myenteric plexus of Auerbach, located between the muscle layers of the muscolaris externa and the submucosal plexus of Meissner.

Microscopic and submicroscopic anatomy

Villi are the motile structures used for absorption. They are supposed to be capable of mixing the lumen content, favoring the absorptive process, and clearing potentially dangerous microorganisms, or antigenic macromolecules.

Scanning electron microscopy provides the most suitable information about the different morphological tridimensional features of *villi*: in the proximal duodenum *villi* are constituted of mucosal ridges, often convoluted (Fig. 1); in the jejunum *villi* acquire the more typical aspect of leaves or tongues or fingers (Fig. 2); in the distal jejunum and ileum *villi* are mostly fingerlike (Fig. 3). Hormonal factors and growth factors are responsible for the different morphology; when a proximal segment is transplanted distally, it acquires all the characteristics of distal mucosa and vice versa. Whether there is any correlation with function is unknown. The surface of *villi* is crossed by shallow furrows; these are due to the contraction of muscolaris mucosae. During absorption *villi* become swollen and their surface becomes smooth.

The tridimensional structure of the enterocytes is observable in artifactual fractures of *villi* (Fig. 4); enterocytes appear as tall columnar or clubbed cells with an apical brush surface covered by *microvilli*, approximately 1 μm in height. On the luminal surface the polygonal profiles of the enterocytes are clearly visible. The basal portion of the enterocytes extends in pseudopodes which attest the ability of these cells to migrate along the wall of *villi*. The **epithelial lining** has a rapid **turnover**, which guarantees an equilibrium between cell proliferation and cell loss. The proliferative zone is situated at the lower half portion of crypts: stem cells become committed to a particular way of differentiation, i.e., into absorptive cells or mucous cells or endocrine cells. Immature, committed cells differentiate during the migration towards the villus tip; they become specialized starting from

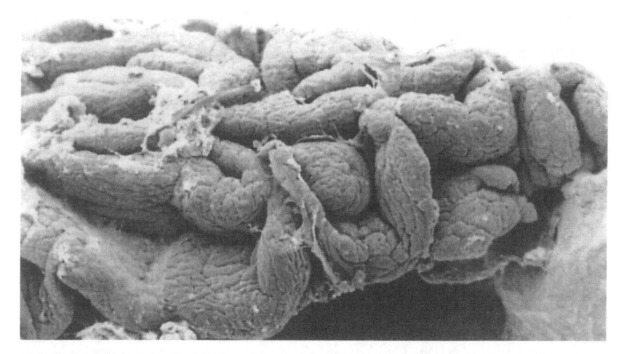

Fig. 1. Proximal duodenum: endoscopic biopsy. The mucosal architecture is constituted by ridges and convolutions (scanning electron microscopy, x 160)

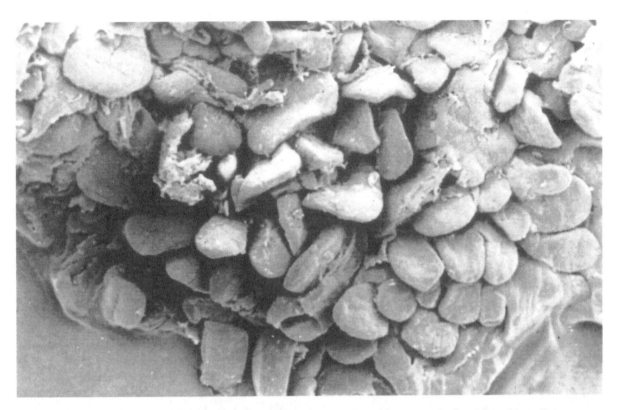

Fig. 2. Jejunum: endoscopic biopsy. The mucosal architecture is constituted by tongue, leaf and fingerlike *villi* (scanning electron microscopy, x 130)

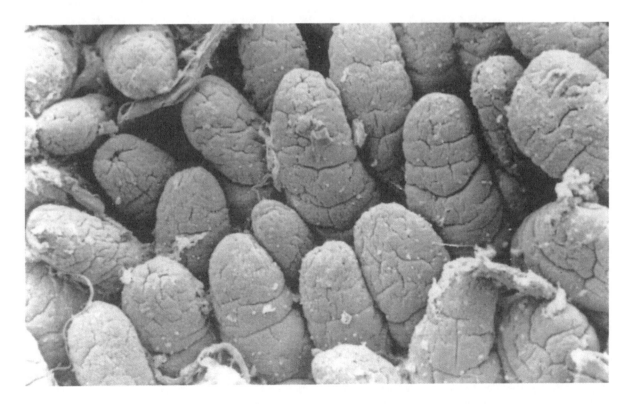

Fig. 3. Distal small bowel: endoscopic biopsy. The mucosal architecture is constituted by fingerlike *villi* (scanning electron microscopy, x 400)

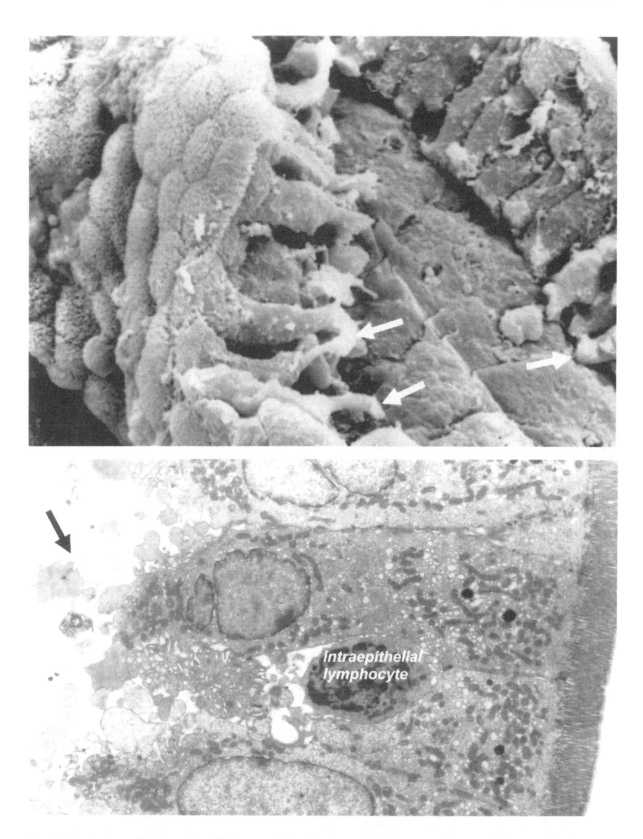

Fig. 4. Jejunal mucosa. *Top*: an artifactually fractured villus shows two rows of enterocytes on a naked portion of villus core. The enterocyte basal portions show pseudopodes (*arrows*); the apical portions shows polygonal outlines and are covered by *microvilli* (scanning electron microscopy, x 3,250). *Bottom*: Enterocytes viewed by transmission electron microscopy. Pseudopodes are indicated by *arrow* (x 6,000)

the middle to the apical portion of *villi*. At villous tips cells desquamate into the lumen (approximately 100-200 g of cells per day). In the duodenum and jejunum it takes 5 days for enterocytes to migrate to the apex, in the ileum 3 days. Paneth cells differentiate by migrating in the opposite way, towards the bottom of the crypt; their turnover is slower (25 days).

Proliferation and migration of epithelial cells and of mesenchymal cells surrounding the crypts occur at the same time, demonstrating the close relation between the two compartments.

As concerns the death of senescent enterocytes, it has been recently demonstrated in experimental animals that enterocytes undergo a programmed cell death or apoptosis. In fact, macrophages phagocytose the basal cytoplasm and the nucleus of senescent cells, while apical cytoplasm and *microvilli* are extruded later in the lumen when other cells have replaced them. This guarantees the integrity of the mucosal barrier. Similar mechanisms of extrusion have been observed in humans as well (author unpublished data) (Fig.5).

The epithelial lining

The cell population of the epithelial lining of the *villi* and crypts is constituted by: enterocytes, or absorptive cells; goblet cells, or mucous cells; Paneth cells, and endocrine cells. The submicroscopic structure of the epithelial lining has been defined by **transmission electron microscopy** (TEM).

Absorptive enterocytes. The high specialization of these cells is evident by TEM. The structures recognizable are related to three main functions: *microvilli* to digestion by plasma membrane enzymes and absorption; cytoplasmic organelles to absorption and transport; and the cytoskeleton to motility (Fig.6).

The cytoskeleton is composed of microfilaments in close relation with the junctional complexes: tonofilaments are 100-Å filaments; they are attached in bundles to desmosomes, connect them, and envelop the portion of the cell beneath the zonula adherens. This provides the cell with steady support for *microvilli* move-

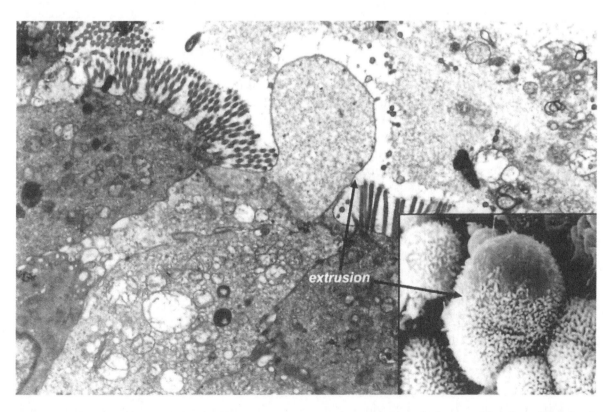

Fig. 5. Jejunal mucosa: the apical portion of a senescent enterocyte is extruded into the lumen, while other cells replace it (transmission electron microscopy, x 13,000). *Inset*: cell extrusion viewed by scanning electron microscopy (x 5,000)

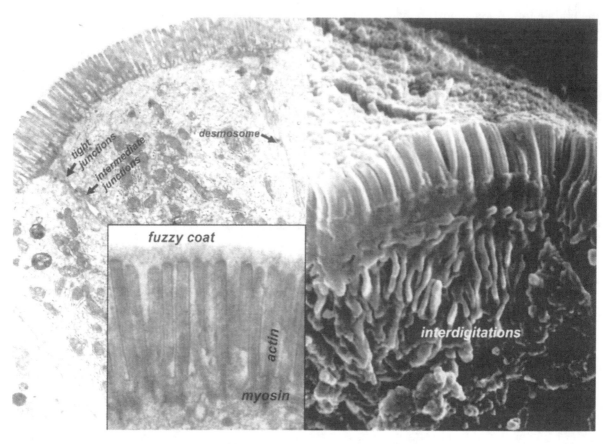

Fig. 6. Jejunal mucosa. *Left*: apical portion of enterocytes and junctional complexes. *Inset*: detail of cytoskeleton (transmission electron microscopy, x 8,600 and x 30,000, respectively. *Right*: tridimensional view of surface and lateral portion of an enterocyte (scanning electron microscopy, x 12,000)

ment. In fact, along the microvillar axis 70-Å F-actin microfilaments are visible. They are anchored to each other and to the lateral inner membrane of the *microvilli* by protein bridges; they extend from microvillus tips to the terminal web. This latter structure is recognizable on the apical cytoplasm and is constituted by a mesh of microfilaments attached to the intermediate junctions; among these, myosin molecules have been demonstrated by immunocytochemistry. The actin-myosin interaction allows the *microvilli* movement. The microvillar motility is considered important for absorption, allowing the mixing of the nutrients which keep in contact with the enterocytes.

Microvilli have specialized membranes capable of both digestion and absorption of nutrients. The outer membrane of the *microvilli* of mature enterocytes, i.e., enterocytes of the mean lateral surface of *villi*, is provided with: (a) a fuzzy coat, constituted by the external projection of the hydrophilic membrane of glycoproteins; pancreatic enzymes are also found entrapped in the fuzzy coat; (b) digestive enzymes such as enterokinase, which activates pancreatic trypsinogen, and enzymes to terminate carbohydrate and protein digestion – disaccharidases (maltase, sucrase-isomaltase, lactase) and peptidases; (c) receptors for selective absorption such as intrinsic factor and carrier proteins which allow the transport of the final products of digestion through the plasma membrane of the enterocyte. Two types of transport are described: active and passive. In normal conditions nutrient transport takes place in the duodenum and jejunum. Ileum absorbs all nutrients as a vicarious function in patients with jejunal resection. In contrast, absorption of vitamin B_{12} and bile salts only takes place in the ileum.

The factors that influence intestinal absorption are still under investigation. Three functions are now taken into consideration as playing a role in absorption: extension of the absorptive surface, intraluminal mixing, and propulsive motility. Absorption is more likely to integrate all three.

Recently a functional structure has been recognized which seems to be crucial for absorptive function even if not detectable with morphological techniques: the so-called *unstirred layer*. This name derives from the consideration that the fluid adjacent to the static surface is not stirred and creates a barrier to the diffusion of solutes. The mixing of the luminal content due to *villi* and *microvilli* make the unstirred layer thinner, thus allowing and favoring absorption.

Mixing of the intervillar luminal content is also necessary for solutes to reach the lateral surfaces of *villi* rapidly and be absorbed.

Lipids have to be emulsified in micelles to become hydrophilic and pass the unstirred layer barrier. The products of triglyceride digestion cross the plasma membrane and are soluted in the cytoplasm bound to the fatty acid binding protein (FABP). In the smooth endoplasmic reticulum triglycerides are re-synthesized. In the RER triglycerides, cholesterol and phospholipids are incorporated into the chilomicrons in which the protein fraction is represented by apoproteins. By inverse pinocytosis chilomicrons are discharged from the basolateral membrane into the intercellular spaces; then they reach the lymphatic vessels. Mean chain fatty acids are directly transported in the portal blood. The transport of absorbed nutrients is allowed and favored by the capillary network of the villus axis which is close to the basal membrane of the epithelial layer (Fig.7); moreover, endothelial cells have a *fenestrated* plasma membrane.

Paneth cells. They are disposed mainly at the bottom of the crypts. In the apical portion of the

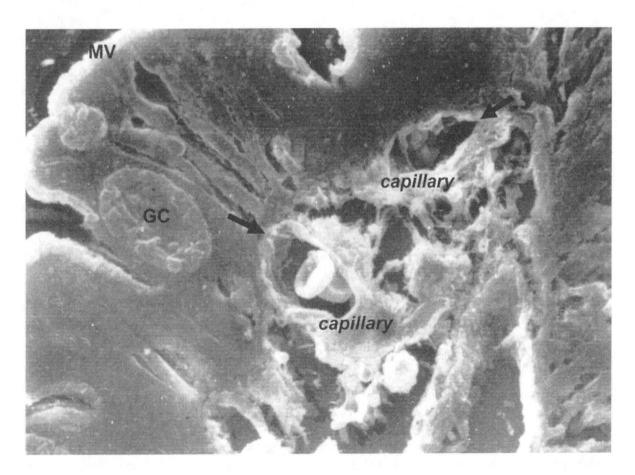

Fig. 7. Jejunal mucosa. The capillary walls are close to the enterocytes (*arrows*); MV, *microvilli*, GC, goblet cell (scanning electron microscopy on semithin section, x 2,500)

The small bowel: structure and function

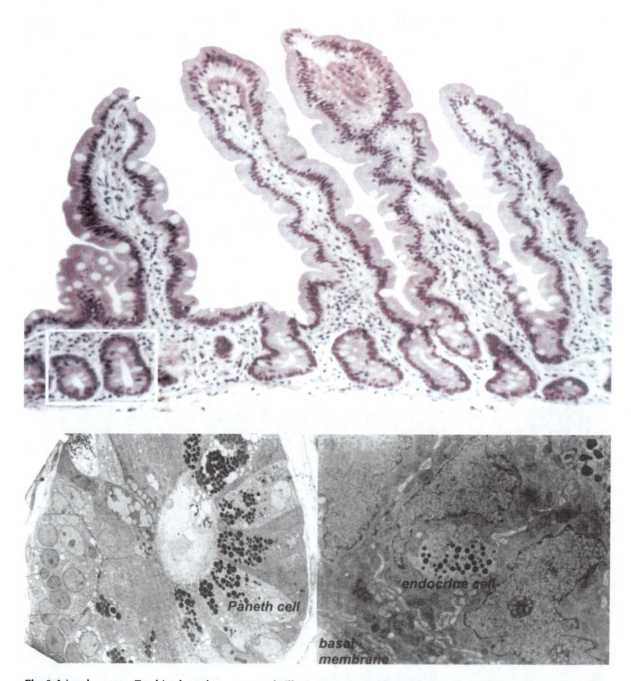

Fig. 8. Jejunal mucosa. *Top*: histology shows a normal villus/crypt ratio. Goblet cells are scattered between epithelial cells of *villi* and crypts (light microscopy, x 300). *Bottom*: Paneth cells in a crypt (*left*, transmission electron microscopy, x 900); endocrine cell in a crypt, with roundish, electron dense small granules (*right*, transmission electron microscopy, x 9,000)

cell, large eosinophilic granules are evident by light microscopy: electron microscopy shows large electron-dense granules. Their function is still unknown. A role in defense mechanisms against bacteria is presumed, as they are able to secrete lysozyme; Paneth cells also contain zinc (Fig.8).

Endocrine cells. In the small intestine they derive from crypt stem cells and are interspersed among the enterocytes of *villi* and crypts. To date, at least 15 types of endocrine cells have been recognized on the basis of morphology of granules or cytochemical or immunocytochemical identification of the secre-

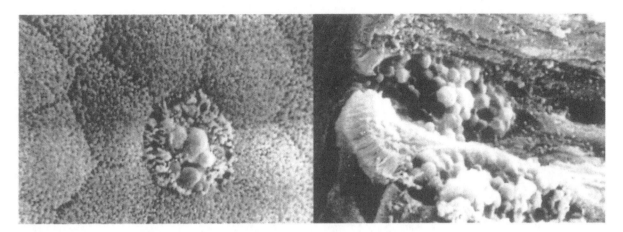

Fig. 9. Luminal surface of goblet cells extruding granules, on the *left*, and lateral surface of goblet cells filled with granules and opening in the lumen, on the *right* (scanning electron microscopy, x 6,500)

tion product (peptides, biogenic amines). Endocrine cells are generally located close to the basal membrane of the epithelium through which they discharge the secretory granules in the lamina propria. The mechanism of action of intestinal peptides is often local, and the cells are more appropriately defined as paracrine instead of endocrine (Fig. 8).

Goblet cells. These cells secrete acid mucins and are supposed to aid the clearance of noxious agents.

Enterocytes and goblet cells form the structural component of the so-called intestinal barrier, which represents the first-line defense of the organism. The impermeability of this barrier is guaranteed by the tight junctions (Fig. 9).

and lymphocytes) are the most represented infiltrating cells of the lamina propria under normal conditions; eosinophil granulocytes are also scattered mainly in the pericryptic zone; neutrophils are not observable under normal conditions. Histiocytes and mast cells are rare; (6) special staining is required to identify mucins; the most common is P.A.S.; (7) as concerns vessels, lymphatics are not visible in fasting in normal conditions; they may be visible during absorption or in pathological condition; and (8) Brunner glands are generally only observed in the duodenum; their function is not well known. They are tubuloalveolar glands extending from the submucosa to mucosa and secreting mucus and bicarbonate.

Histomorphology of the small intestine

When the small intestine mucosa is observed by light microscopy in routinely stained sections (Fig. 8), the parameters which have to be taken into account are mainly: (1) the orientation of the mucosal sample has to be correct, with *villi* and crypts perpendicular to the muscularis mucosae, to avoid a false aspect of atrophy; (2) height of *villi* and crypts and crypt/villus ratio which is 1:3-4 under normal conditions; (3) integrity of the epithelial lining; (4) number (density) of intraepithelial lymphocytes; (5) lamina propria cells: mononuclear cells (plasma cells

Immunocompetent cells of the small intestine

The small intestine exposes the entire surface to the external environment. Its defense mechanism is expressed by lymphoid cells, lymphoepithelial organs and specialized epithelial cells.

Intraepithelial lymphocytes are characteristic, infiltrating T-cells of the small intestine, being rare in stomach and in colon. Their phenotype is mainly CD8 suppressor/cytotoxic. Their density, calculated as number of cells per epithelial area or number of cells related to number of epithelial cells (1:4 in normal conditions), enhances in relation to antigenic stimulation by

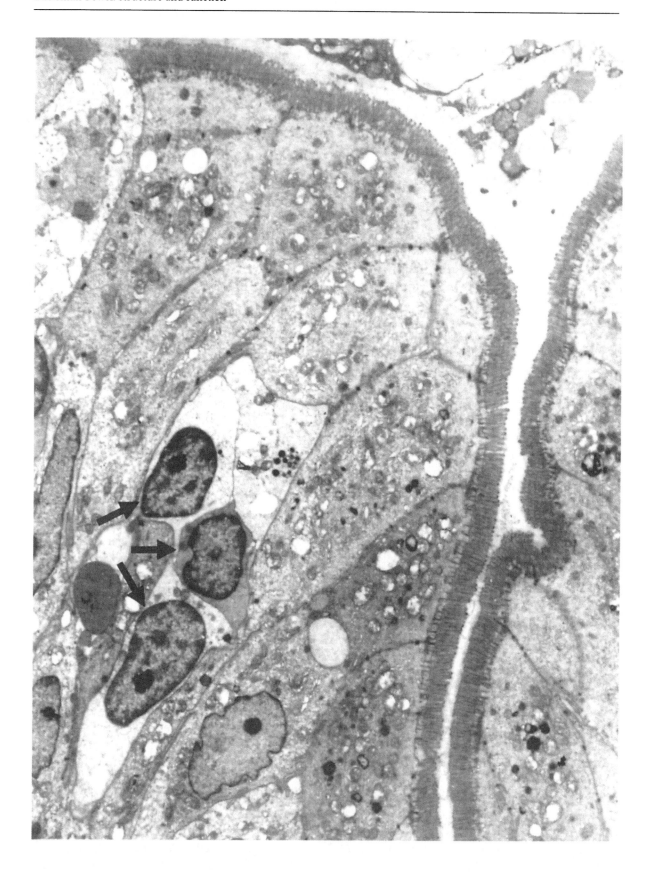

Fig. 10. Jejunal mucosa. Intraepithelial lymphocytes infiltrated between enterocytes (transmission electron microscopy, x 6,000)

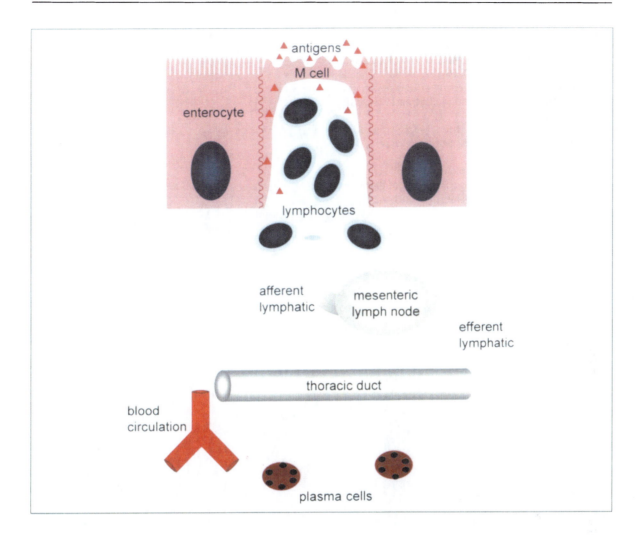

Fig. 11. Mucosal associated lymphoid tissue and M-cell

microorganisms, macromolecules, etc. (Fig. 10). Immunocytochemistry is necessary to characterize them. Plasma cells infiltrate the lamina propria and have a characteristic submicroscopic morphology; the nuclear eterochromatin is clumped. In cytoplasm the RER is expanded, especially in phases of activation and synthesis of immunoglobulins. The type of immunoglobulin secreted is recognizable by immunocytochemistry. Small intestine plasma cells synthesize mainly IgA dimers which bind to a glycoprotein receptor on the basolateral membrane of the epithelial cells, cross the epithelial cell, and are secreted into the lumen bound to the so-called *secretory piece* or component.

Lymphoepithelial organs are constituted by lymphatic follicles located under the epithelial lining; the epithelial cells covering a lymphatic follicle are constituted by normal columnar, absorptive enterocytes and by the so-called M-cells. M-cells are cells located as a bridge between the enterocytes; they have a thin cytoplasm which extends from one cell to another. The surface membrane has microfolds. M-cells are able to transport antigens from the intestinal lumen through the cell and the basolateral membrane in contact with lymphocytes and macrophages; activated T+ and B lymphocytes migrate into afferent lymphatics to mesenteric lymph nodes, from which they enter efferent lymphatics, the thoracic duct, and, finally, the peripheral blood. In the meanwhile, lymphocytes become lymphoblasts which can recirculate back to the site of activation; by this process of *homing*, B lymphoblasts become plasma cells secreting IgA as a specific immunological response (Fig. 11).

Suggested reading

Bonvicini F, Zoli G, Maltarello MC, Bianchi D, Pasquinelli G, Versura P, Gasbarrini G, Laschi R (1985) Clinical applications of scanning electron microscopy in gastrointestinal diseases. Scanning Electron Microsc III: 1279-1294

Fenoglio-Preiser C, Lantz PE, Listrom MB, Davis M, Rilke FO (1989) Gastrointestinal pathology. Raven, New York, pp 167-186

Rubin W (1991) Small intestine: anatomy and structural anomalies. In: Yamada T (ed) Textbook of gastroenterology. Lippincott, Philadelphia, pp 1409-1424

DIAGNOSTIC METHODOLOGIES

Small bowel imaging procedures

Transabdominal ultrasonography

Nuclear tests

Small bowel imaging procedures

D. Regent

Optimizing the timeline of the various available procedures is a major problem when studying the small intestine. Maximum efficiency, rendering the most accurate diagnosis in a minimal time with minimum "aggressiveness" toward the patient and the lowest cost for the community is the goal to reach.

Immutably, imaging procedures are prescribed and cumulate systematically from the so-called "common" exams (plain film of abdomen, ultrasound opacification) to the alledgedly more sophisticated and expensive ones (CT and MRI).

This pattern has several disadvantages, among them the proceedings stretching in time, redundant results, and always higher costs. We will have to adjust our attitudes and options to:
- newcoming techniques, such as enteroscopy
- improving results of current procedures due to imaging enhancement (CT and MRI) and technical developments (high-resolution ultrasound, color Doppler)
- the effective overall cost, the wear and tear on the patient and, most of all, the diagnostic effectiveness

Plain film of the abdomen

Routinely and systematically prescribed, a plain film examination is considered "low cost" and harmless. That might be true for an ambulatory patient, but it certainly is questionable when applied to an intensive care unit patient. This finding will be addressed again in further procedures. The benefit then is poor and the induced expenses unnecessary. It should not be systematically prescribed anymore. Even as an emergency examination, its sensitivity and specificity range at best between 60% and 80 % in occlusion and hollow viscera perforation cases, and the statistical rate drops further in ischemia cases. The plain film of the abdomen is daily and widely outranked by the increased success of CT and ultrasound. Only monitoring a specific pathology can comply with such a poor diagnostic examination (for example, an obstruction syndrome with a favorable course).

Ultrasonography

Performed with strict technical rules by a skilled practitioner, ultrasound can be very useful in bowel loops and mesenteric examinations. But due to practical inconveniences, this procedure is mainly carried out in specialized centers. Under usual conditions, the sensitivity is low and only positive findings are considered.

On the other hand, ultrasound may be valuable in analyzing the different layers of an otherwise detected lesion. High frequency probes (5 or even 7.5 MHz according to anatomical conditions) should then be used. Vascular Doppler imaging has proven its usefulness, especially in inflammatory diseases.

Small intestine opacification techniques

Double-contrast enteroclysis rather than simple barium ingestion should be used for small bowel examination. Whichever method utilized, the small bowel examination should not be employed to screen a general or focal disease. The development of other techniques such as CT and ultrasound leaves small bowel opacification as a second-intention examination. Even well-performed, one has to be aware of:
- patient fatigue, especially the inconvenience of the tube positioning in enteroclysis
- the difficulty in performing and palpating pelvic loops on slender and hyposthenic individuals
- irradiation
- cost, considering the personnel and equipment immobilization

It is an "indirect" visualization method which only allows an accurate overview of the parietal lesion extension and the mechanical effects.

First-intention small bowel examinations are mainly conducted to monitor Crohn's disease; mainly its mechanical repercussions and the lesion length, secondary post-surgical adhesions, and internal, hernia-related complications.

Very specific indications, such as Meckel's diverticulum complications, can still persist.

For tumorous lesions, enteroclysis remains the first diagnostic tool in two circumstances:
- in "napkin ring" adenocarcinoma characterized by a very short stenosis (1 to 3 cm) centered on a very narrow channel, less than 1 cm in diameter
- for small lesions of the superficial layers of the intestinal wall, in lymphomatous superficial nodules, carcinoid tumors, and inflammatory and adenomatous polyps

CT imaging

CT scan has been a major and well-founded development in digestive tract radiology over the past 5 years.

Fast rotational scans, high-resolution images (512 x 512 matrix), thin slices (5 mm), and data processing (multiplanar reformations) lead to a better knowledge of the normal appearance as well as the pathological anatomy in mesenteric and intestinal disorders. The efficiency of CT has been proven in acute abdomen studies, escpecially obstructions, perforations, and ischemia. Major benefits were also brought up in small bowel inflammatory and tumoral pathology.

The accessibility to CT scans, the technical mastery of the radiologists and the clinical management partners (surgeons, endoscopic medical teams) should confirm its prevailing role as a first-intention examination.

A few technical basics need to be remembered, though:
- initial scan, thick and spaced slices in order to spot the area of interest, determined by peritoneal fat infiltration and soft tissue opacity areas
- thin slice scanning of the suspected areas enhanced through intravenous iodine administration
- careful look at the enhanced wall-thickened area to differentiate "circumferential submucosal edema", typical of acute parietal lesions (inflammatory, infectious or ischemic) from a tumoral process
- precise study of the serous interface to find "spicular infiltration" images, attesting an inflammatory (Crohn's diasease) or a tumoral process

Besides the search for a deep abscess (sometimes hard to distinguish from a dilated loop), oral opacification (barium or water-soluble contrast) is no longer necessary.

On the other hand, water-filled and dilated loops (whether in obstruction cases or from swallowing water, or even water enteroclysis) can be a great help in parietal lesion analysis.

The current real-time reformation possibilities let us foresee further developments in scanning techniques, such as coronal views, offering better interpretation in many pathologies.

Magnetic resonance imaging

Slow scanning in classic MRI was not of much service to the study of visceral developments,

but recent major improvements now permit short scanning times, more appropriate to an older or sick patient's breath-holding capability. Two types of sequences are available:
- fast T1-weighted gradient echo (Turbo FLASH, FMPSPGR), allowing dynamic studies by repeating on demand a 15- to 20-s-long slice batch.
- more recently, hyper T2 "single shot" sequences, allowing thin slices (7 to 50 mm or more) in a 1- to 5-s scan time and offering real entero-MRI coronal and oblique views. With more predictable improvements, MRI will easily replace CT, which will do away with irradiation and nephrotoxic iodine injections.

Angiography

Today, diagnostic angiography plays a very limited role in intestinal and mesenteric investigations. It is restricted to:
- diagnosis of hemorrhagic lesions that have not been detected by other procedures
- diagnosis of acute or chronic ischemic lesions, followed by an immediate therapeutic modality

These indications are limited to:
- occlusion of the superior mesenteric artery and its branches, occurring within a time period allowing thombolysis or thromboaspiration
- proximal stenosis of the superior mesenteric artery, when transluminal angioplasty is planned

Conclusion

The feasibility of small intestine "virtual endoscopy" can be expected either from CT or entero-MR images.

Nevertheless, difficulties in current implementation of the technique should be feared, because correct results are dependent on a strictly homogeneous endoluminal content which seems hard to obtain even with the enteroclysis of water, contrast medium, or gas.

Suggested reading

Amberg JR (1994) Small bowel examination: overview. In: Freeny PC, Stevenson GW, Margulis AR, Burkenneís (eds) Alimentary tract radiology, 5th edn. Mosby, St Louis, pp 689-691

Brooke Jeffrey R, Walls PW (1996) CT and sonography of the acute abdomen, 2nd edn, Lippincott-Raven, Philadelphia, pp 256-314

Vecchioli A, De Franco A, Maresca G, Gore RM (1994) Small bowel-cross sectorial imaging. In: Gore RM, Levine MS, Laufer I (eds) Textbook of gastrointestinal radiology. Saunders Philadelphia, pp 304-315

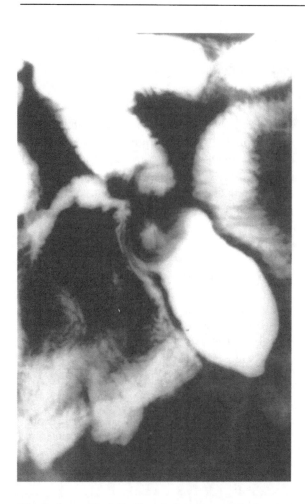

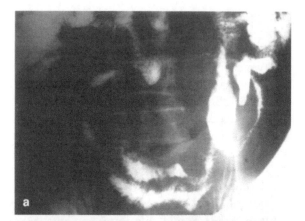
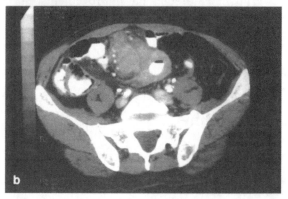

Fig. 1. *Large Meckel's diverticulum.* Large blind-ended non-folded sac arising from the antimesenteric border of terminal ileum. Ulceration at the ileal junction is clearly shown

Fig. 2. *NH lymphoma.* **a** CT. Segmental, circumferential thickening of ileum wall with homogeneous mass of the mesentery. Absence of mechanical obstruction showing that there is no retracting stroma-reaction fibrosis. **b** Small bowel follow-through. Opacification shows only indirect signs of lymphomatous infiltration of intestinal wall: rigid aspect of the lumen borders and separation from adjoining bowel loops

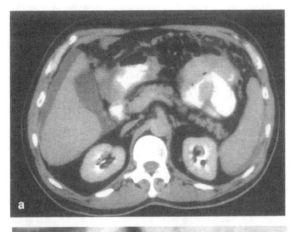
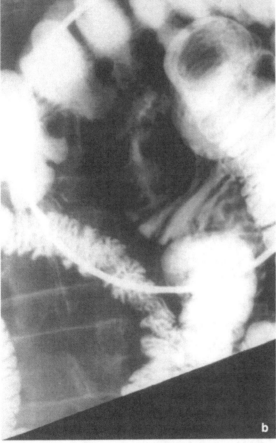

Fig. 3. *Stenosing adenocarcinoma of the first jejunal loop with peritoneal carcinomatosis.* **a** CT. Narrowed stenosis of the jejunal lumen due to a huge mass infiltrating the proximal mesentery. **b** Enteroclysis only identifies the stenosing "apple-core" lesion with upper mechanical dilation with difficulty

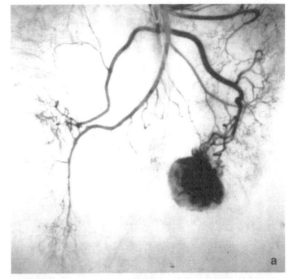
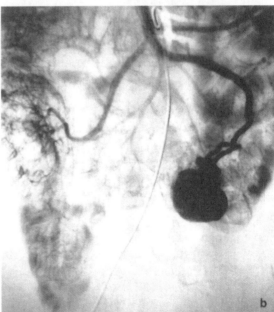

Fig. 4. *Large exoluminal leiomyoma causing repeated gastro-intestinal hemorrhage.* **a** SMA selective angiography. Arterial phase. Large heterogeneous hypervascular ileal tumor. The lesion is characterized by its polycyclic, well-circumscribed shape. **b** Venous phase. Dilated superior mesenteric vein due to intratumorous arteriovenous shunting determining blood hyperflow rate

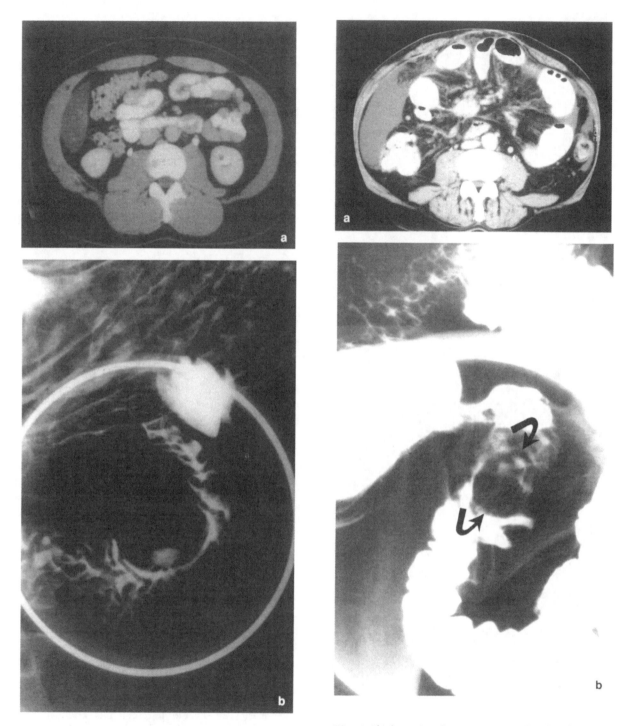

Fig. 5. *Small leiomyoma of the first jejunal loop.* **a** CT. Small, rounded tumor next to the Treitz angle with central ulceration. **b** Central ulceration is well seen at the top of the rounded endoluminal graving tumor

Fig. 6. *Ileal carcinoid tumor.* **a** Spiculated soft tissue mesenteric mass pathognomonic of carcinoid tumors. **b** Submucosa nodular lesions of a distal ileum loop corresponding to initial carcinoid lesion

Atlas of Enteroscopy

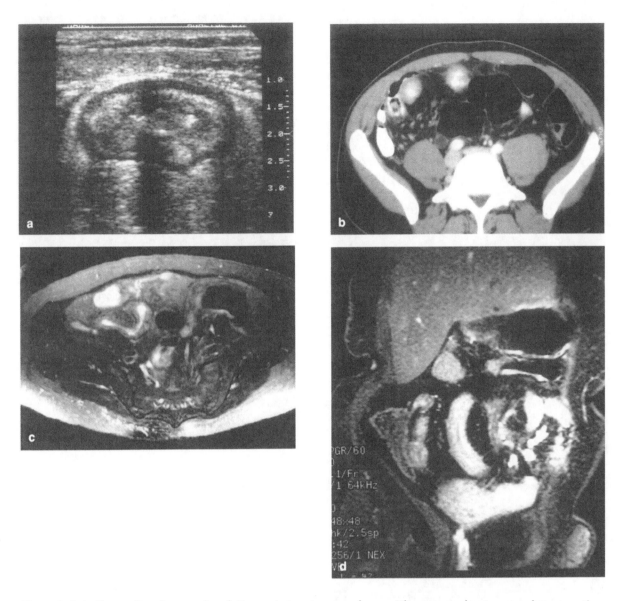

Fig. 7. *Crohn's disease. Complementarity of diagnostic imaging procedures.* **a** Ultrasonography: transversal cross section. Thickened and hyperechoic mesentery (*bottom*). Multiple transmural deep ulcers are well demonstrated. **b** CT. Circular thickening of intestinal wall with mesenteric fibrofatty proliferation and spikes of perivascular fibrosis along the mesenteric border "comb sign". **c** Axial FSE slice (MRI). T2-weighted image shows the ileal lumen's liquid content. **d** Coronal view. Fast T1-weighted gradient echo, along with fat saturation and gadolinium injection. Good view of the fibrous spiculations along the vascular tracks on the mesenteric side (comb sign)

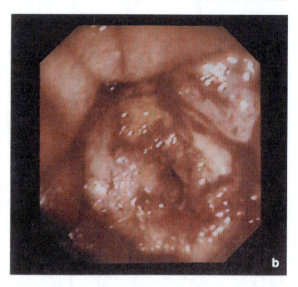

Fig. 9. *Hemorrhagic adenomatous ileal polyp.* Selective SMA arteriogram. A 15-mm hypervascularized node in the ileal lumen

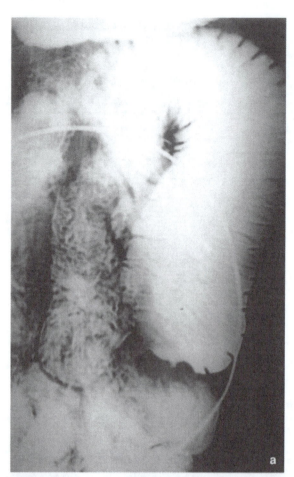

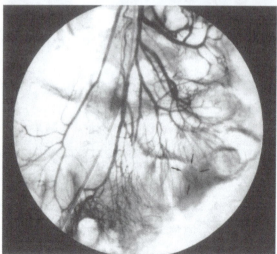

Fig. 8. *Short "napkin ring" stenosing adenocarcinoma.* **a.** Enteroclysis remains the most efficient tool in diagnosing this particuliar short-length stenosing adenocarcinoma. **b** Enteroscopic aspect of the tumorous "diaphragm" and its narrow central orifice

Transabdominal ultrasonography

V. Arienti

In the past, because of its inability to penetrate gas, ultrasonography (US) was considered a useless method for studying the gastrointestinal tract. In more recent years, thanks to the technological improvement of ultrasonographic instruments and to the greater attention of researchers, the ultrasonographic findings of some intestinal pathologies have been described. Different ultrasonographic approaches and modalities have been proposed such as conventional or transabdominal, endoscopic, transrectal, hydrocolonic and Doppler and color-Doppler ultrasonography. Today the ultrasonographic method commonly employed in the evaluation of small bowel pathologies is transabdominal ultrasound, utilizing 3.5, 5, and 7 MHz linear or convex probes, with the help, in some cases, of the Doppler and color-Doppler modality.

Normal aspects

The normal bowel wall thickness is generally less than 3 mm, and its US aspect varies greatly in relation to its luminal content (gas, liquid or *ingesta*). If gas is prevailing, the typical ultrasonographic feature is characterized by hyperechoic curved lines with partial posterior acoustic shadow; if the liquid content prevails, this is visualized as anechoic areas containing hyperechoic "spots"; finally, *ingesta* are represented as moving hypoechoic areas. The movement makes it possible to distinguish *ingesta* from lymphadenopathies. The small bowel and colon can be recognized thanks to the different aspect of *valvulae conniventes,* in the *ileum,* and to the constant presence of gas in the colon.

Utilizing 5 and 7 MHz linear or convex probes, it is sometimes possible to visualize the stratification of the intestinal wall, consisting of five layers: the first, hyperechoic, represents the *interface* lumen/mucosal surface; the second, hypoechoic, the mucosa; the third, hyperechoic, the submucosa; the fourth, hypoechoic, the *muscularis propria* and the fifth, hyperechoic, the serosa and the adjacent fat tissue. The stratification of the US aspect is visible in the small bowel and colon only in pathological conditions, while in the esophagus, stomach and rectum it can also be seen in normal conditions.

Pathological aspects

Transcutaneous ultrasonography can reveal various intestinal diseases; most of them have the same ultrasonographic finding characterized by an echogenic center, which represents the intestinal lumen, and an echo-poor halo of variable thickness, which represents the thickened bowel wall. This US sign is defined using different terms: "target," "cockade" or "bull's-eye," in transversal section; "sandwich" or "pseudokidney," in longitudinal section, has a poor correlation with the etiological nature of the disease. In fact, it can occur in several pathologic conditions such as muscular hypertrophy, hemorrhage, ischemia, inflammation and neoplasm. Bowel-wall thickening represents the typical, most frequent US finding in diseases of the gut; associated US abnormalities are the modifications of luminal content and peristalsis, the presence of fluid collections in the abdominal cavity, abscesses, fistulas and mesenteric fibro-fatty proliferation.

The main indications of transcutaneous ultrasonography in small bowel disease are Crohn's disease, bacterial, necrotizing, pseudomembranous and radiation enteritis, acute ischemia, celiac and Whipple's diseases and tumors (Table 1). A sonographic diagnosis of obstructed afferent loop is visible as a distended fluid-filled segment with a multilayered wall and few mucosal folds.

Table 1. US of small bowel (indications)

• Crohn's disease	• Radiation enteritis
• Bacterial enteritis	• Acute ischemia
• Necrotizing enteritis	• Celiac disease
• Pseudomembranous enteritis	• Whipple's disease
	• Tumors

A great deal of information can be obtained by ultrasonography in patients with **Crohn's disease**. The most frequent ultrasonographic finding is the transmural bowel wall thickening, which is the result of the combination of inflammatory cell infiltration, edema and fibrosis. Other manifestations of Crohn's disease which can be demonstrated by ultrasound are dilated pre-stenotic loops, conglomeration of bowel loops, fluid-filled loops, luminal narrowing, mesenteric proliferation, abscesses and fistulas (Table 2).

Table 2. Crohn's disease (US findings)

• Transmural bowel-wall thickening	• Fluid-filled loops
	• Luminal narrowing
• Dilated pre-stenotic loops	• Mesenteric proliferation
• Conglomeration	• Abscesses and fistulas

The sensitivity, specificity and overall accuracy of ultrasound in the diagnosis of Crohn's disease are about 90%; the sensitivity and specificity of indium-scan and US in detecting X-ray defined lesions are similar and bowel-wall thickening is significantly related to scintigraphic intensity of emission. Ultrasonography has the same accuracy as computed tomography in detecting abdominal or intra-abdominal abscesses, while computed tomography is superior in cases of retroperitoneal or perianal abscesses. Enteroenteric fistulas are difficult to visualize; in contrast, enterovescical fistulas are easily recognizable. Transcutaneous ultrasonography has been proposed as the primary screening method in suspected cases and in the detection of post-surgical recurrences; its main applications are represented by the possibility of assessing the location and extent of the disease, detecting the possible complications, following patients, evaluating the response to medical treatment, and differentiating Crohn's disease from ulcerative colitis and tumors (Table 3).

Table 3. Crohn's disease (US role)

• Primary screening (?)	• Follow-up
• Disease assessment	• Response to treatment
– location	• Differential diagnosis
– extent	– other enteritis
– activity	– ulcerative colitis
• Complications	– appendicitis, adnexitis
• Post-surgical recurrences	– tumors

Pronounced bowel-wall thickness, transmural involvement of the bowel wall, ileal localization, segmental distribution and the presence of complications (abscesses, fistulas and mesenterial proliferation) are all findings in favor of Crohn's disease with respect to ulcerative colitis. A gradual increase of thickness in the bowel wall, symmetrical layers and a lumen in the central position suggest an inflammatory condition and exclude tumors, with the exception of lymphoma. By means of Doppler ultrasound it is possible to detect a higher mean flow velocity in portal and mesenteric veins and a significantly lower resistance index in superior mesenteric arteries in patients with active inflammatory disease with respect to inactive disease and controls. Color Doppler ultrasonography permits an accurate evaluation of vascular flow in the bowel wall and also precise positioning of sample volume with quantitative evaluation of the Doppler wave.

Bacterial enteritis due to *Yersinia enterocolitica* or *Staphylococcus* has US aspects similar to Crohn's disease, i.e., ileal and cecal wall thickening. Therefore, the US picture must be correlated with the clinical evaluation. In the case of bacterial enteritis the clinical pattern is acute, while in Crohn's disease this US aspect is associated with slight-moderate clinical activity. Although bacteriologic, serologic, radiographic and endoscopic confirmation is necessary, sonography can be useful for the detection of *Y. enterocolitica* or *Staphylococcus* acute terminal ileitis.

In **necrotizing enteritis**, caused by the beta-toxin of *Clostridium perfringens*, US can demonstrate bowel-wall thickening, gaseous distension, fluid-filled loops, and air in the portal venous system.

The ultrasonographic diagnosis of **pseudomembranous enterocolitis** is based on features of superficial, moderate-to-marked wall thickening, ascites in a patient with diarrhea and a history of antibiotic therapy.

Radiation enteritis is frequent in the female sex because of radiation therapies for gynecological tumors. The ultrasonographic pattern is characterized by conglomerated and dilated loops, fluid-filled luminal content, hyperperistalsis, reduction of *valvulae conniventes*, slight bowel-wall thickening, short stenotic tracts and mesenteric hypertrophy.

Acute intestinal ischemia is associated with high mortality, and improvement of the unfavorable prognosis appears possible if the diagnosis is made early enough. Ultrasonography can detect ischemic changes in the intestinal wall: bowel-wall thickening, intramural air ("*pneumatous intestinalis*"), free liquid, free air, possibly also air in the portal venous system, stenotic mesenteric vessels by means of duplex Doppler sonography, absence of or barely visible color Doppler flow. Duplex and color Doppler flow US are helpful in differentiating between ischemic and inflammatory bowel-wall thickening.

The malabsorption syndromes principally investigated in recent years by ultrasonography, are celiac and Whipple's diseases.

In **coeliac disease** ultrasonography only shows indirect signs of malabsorption: fluid-filled loops, abnormal meteorism, hyperperistalsis, absence of wall thickening and mesenteric proliferation. Doppler sonography can reveal an increase in both mean flow velocity and end-diastolic velocity and a reduction in pulsatility index in untreated compared with treated patients.

Whipple's disease is a rare, multiorgan disease that typically involves the small intestine and causes malabsorption. Abdominal ultrasonography shows dilated and thickened loops and abdominal lymph nodes which are considerably increased in volume and markedly hyperechoic; this latter aspect would suggest Whipple's disease and is linked to the accumulation of fats.

Small intestinal **tumors** are difficult to visualize. As mentioned above, when a "target pattern" is recognized, it is possible to differentiate neoplasms from benign inflammatory lesions. A malignancy pattern is characterized by an abrupt transition from the normal wall to the thickened pathological tract, asymmetry of the layers and a lumen in an eccentric position. Lymphoma represents the only exception to this rule, because it has a US pattern similar to the inflammatory diseases. Malignancy lesions are usually diagnosed by means of endoscopy and barium studies. Fine-needle aspiration-biopsy should be regarded as an integral part of US examination, and the indications for an ultrasound study, including biopsy, are equivocal barium studies and false-negative endoscopically guided biopsy, especially in cases of cancers infiltrating the submucous layers or an intestinal mass of undetermined nature. The overall diagnostic accuracy of fine-needle aspiration biopsy is about 90%. The main contraindication, apart from coagulation defects, is the puncture of distended loops.

Conclusions

Abdominal ultrasound is frequently the first investigation in patients with various abdominal symptoms, and there is a growing appreciation of its value in a wide range of gastrointestinal disorders. Thanks to its characteristics - quick, safe, readily available, non-invasive - it is now considered the primary diagnostic method in specific conditions; for example, in cases of acute pain in the right lower quadrant, US permits the differential diagnosis between the three most frequent pathologies, i.e. appendicitis, terminal ileitis, right ovarian pathology. In many cases, ultrasound can be promptly diagnostic of bowel pathology; otherwise, it can exclude or identify possible diseases, suggesting the most appropriate sequences of diagnostic investigation. The principal limitation of this method is represented by the experience of the examiner. To obtain high diagnostic results, especially in small bowel pathology, it is indispensable to correlate the ultrasonographic features with the clinical data.

Suggested reading

Arienti V, Califano C, Brusco G, Boriani L, Biagi F, Sama MG, Sottili S, Domanico A, Corazza GR, Gasbarrini G (1996) Doppler ultrasonographic evaluation of splanchnic blood flow in coeliac disease. Gut 39:369-373

Brignola C, Belloli C, Iannone P, De Simone G, Corbelli C, Levorato M, Arienti V, Boriani L, Gionchetti P, et al (1993) Comparison of scintigraphy with indium-111 leukocyte scan and ultrasonography in assessment of X-ray-demonstrated lesions of Crohn's disease. Dig Dis Sci 38:433-437

Schwerk WB, Beckh K, Raith M (1992) A prospective evaluation of high resolution sonography in the diagnosis of inflammatory bowel disease. Eur J Gastroenterol Hepatol 4:173-182

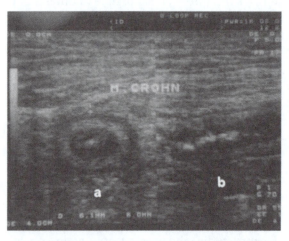

Fig. 1. "Target," "cockade" or "bull's-eye" US aspect visualized in transversal section (**a**) and "sandwich" or "pseudokidney" US aspect visualized in longitudinal section (**b**)

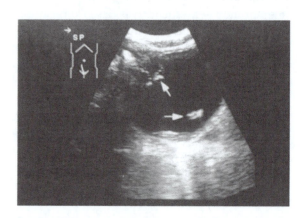

Fig. 2. Spilling (*arrows*) of enteric content into the bladder

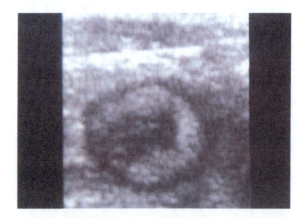

Fig. 3. Ileal localization of Crohn's disease with symmetrical layers and lumen in the central position

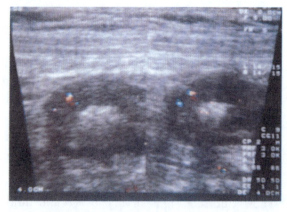

Fig. 4. Presence of color Doppler signals in an inflamed, thickened bowel wall

Atlas of Enteroscopy

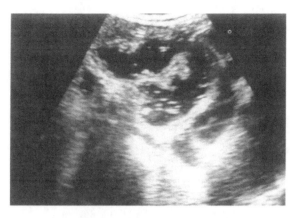

Fig. 5. Conglomerated and dilated, fluid-filled loops in radiation enteritis

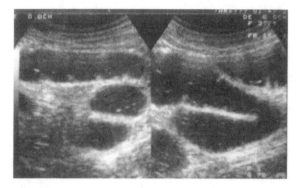

Fig. 6. Fluid-filled, distended loops in a patient with celiac disease

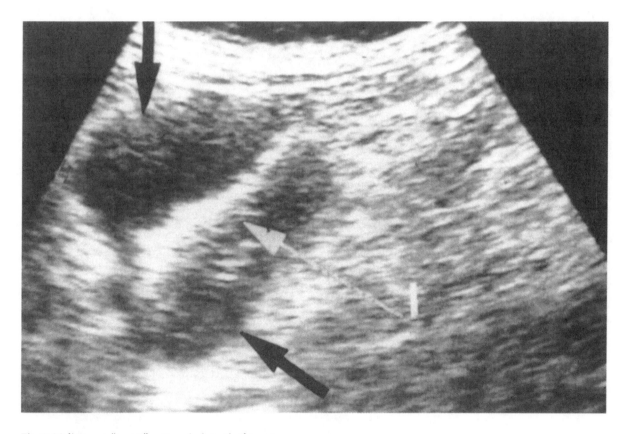

Fig. 7. Malignancy "target" pattern in intestinal tumor

Nuclear tests

G. Sciarretta, A. Furno

The small bowel is difficult to explore by invasive techniques because of its anatomical position and loop conformation; therefore, a noninvasive imaging examination like scintigraphy may be particularly useful.

Since the 1970s 111-indium-labeled leukocytes or granulocytes have been successfully employed to detect inflammation by means of scintigraphy that has been validated in assessing the site, extent and activity in inflammatory bowel diseases (IBD) such as ulcerative colitis and Crohn's disease (CD).

More recently, white cells have been labeled with technetium-99m hexamethyl propylene amine oxime, ^{99m}Tc-HMPAO (Ceretec-Amersham Int.) with better images, lower radiation burden and a more readily availabile radiocompound. Clinical studies on CD have shown that the ^{99m}Tc-HMPAO white cell scan has a high accuracy for the assessment of inflammatory activity; it gives exact information about the site, extent and possible complications such as abscesses and fistulas; moreover, it allows follow-up of the disease after medical or surgical treatment.

From the clinical studies published on CD patients we can state that ^{99m}Tc-HMPAO white cell scan, if the cellular fraction separation and labelling are correctly performed, can give an answer to the following questions:
1. Wheter or not small bowel loops are involved in active inflammation in CD or in other diseases with an inflammatory component.
2. The site and extent of inflammation.
3. The degree of inflammation according to a grading score established on the scintigraphic image intensity that is very well correlated with the histological inflammatory activity.
4. The possible presence of CD complications.
5. The evaluation of CD activity after treatment.

It must be underlined that the ^{99m}Tc-HMPAO white cell scan can show inflammation, but it cannot establish an exact diagnosis. Other invasive examinations such as endoscopy and histology must still be done.

Another interesting clinical use of the ^{99m}Tc-HMPAO white cell scan is the early study of patients with a low probability of IBD; in these cases the technique proved to have a high diagnostic accuracy for detecting active inflammation, thus allowing more invasive tests to be omitted in cases with a negative scan.

Bleeding of the small bowel represents a clinical problem when endoscopic or radiological techniques fail to show the cause. Meckel's diverticulum may cause bleeding in children, but is uncommon in adults; it has an incidence of 1.5%-2%, but bleeding occurs only in those with ectopic gastric mucosa in the diverticulum (5%-15% overall).

^{99m}Tc-pertechnetate scintigraphy has been extensively used to detect ectopic gastric mucosa because of its capability of being concentrated by gastric mucosa regardless of the presence or absence of parietal cells. The technique is simple and safe and 75%-100% sensitivity values have been reported. Pentagastrin given subcutaneously 15 min before ^{99m}Tc-pertechnetate administration may enhance uptake by the diverticulum. Positive scans show a persistent area of uptake usually in the right mid-abdomen.

In adults, other causes of bleeding are to be considered, so ^{99m}Tc in-vivo-labelled red blood cells can offer an answer in cases where the origin in the small bowel is unknown. After intravenous radionuclide administration, serial abdominal images are taken for 24 h. This technique can detect the site of bleeding with a flow of at least 0.3 ml/min.

Suggested reading

Berquist TH, Nolan NG, Stephens DH, Carlson HC (1976) Specificity of 99mTc pertechnetate in scintigraphy diagnosis of Meckel's diverticulum: review of 100 cases. J Nucl Med 17: 465-469

Malcolm PN, Bearcroft CP, Pratt PG, Rampton DS, Garvie NW (1994) Technetium-99m hexamethylpropylene amine oxime labelled leucocyte scanning in the initial diagnosis of Crohn's disease. Br J Radiol 67: 964-968

Sciarretta G, Furno A, Mazzoni M, Basile C, Malaguti P (1993) Technetium-99m hexamethyl propylene amine oxime granulocyte scintigraphy in Crohn's disease: diagnostic and clinical relevance. Gut 34: 1364-1369

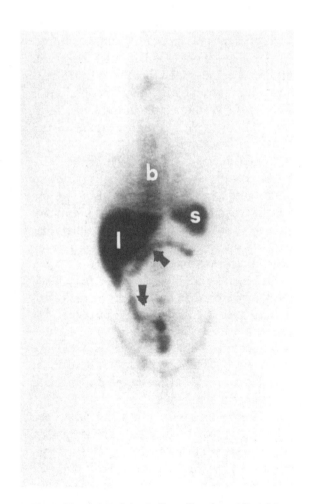

Fig. 1. Normal activity in liver (l), spleen (s) and bone-marrow (b). Active CD in jejunum and proximal ileum (*arrows*)

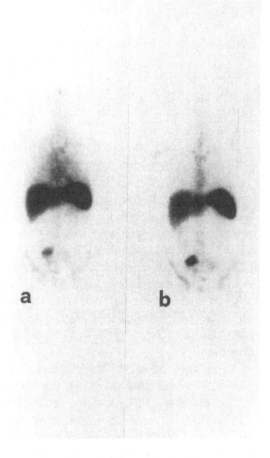

Fig. 2. Focal white blood cells accumulation in CD patient at 2 h (**a**). Also evident in the same position at late 24 h image (**b**). Scintigraphic pattern suggesting an abscess complication

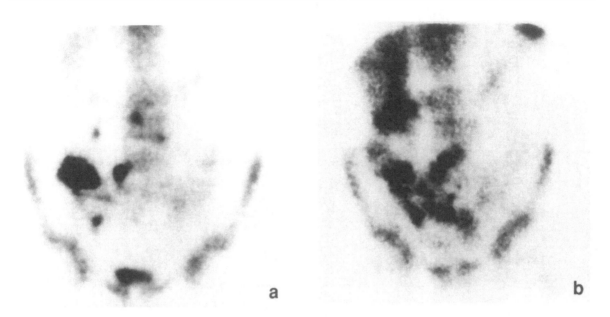

Fig. 3. Early (**a**) and late (**b**) images of enteroenteric fistulas in a small bowel CD patient

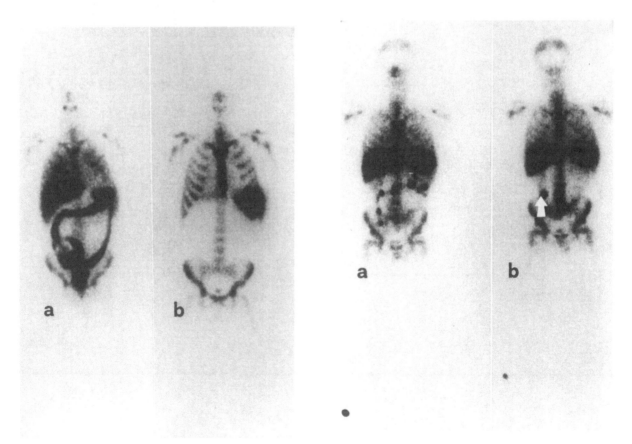

Fig. 4. Ileum and colon CD before (**a**) and after 2 years treatment with steroids and azathioprine (**b**). Complete remission of inflammation is observed

Fig. 5. Segmentary involvement of jejunum and ileum by CD (**a**). After distal ileum resection and stricturoplasty an anastomotic recurrence (*arrow*) is clearly shown (**b**)

ENTEROSCOPY

Sonde enteroscopy

Push enteroscopy

Intraoperative enteroscopy

Laparoscopically assisted enteroscopy

Sonde enteroscopy

J.F. MacKenzie

Flexible endoscopy of the gastrointestinal tract, using fiberoptic techniques and more recently silicon chip technology, has allowed easy visual access to the inside of the upper and lower gastrointestinal tract. From above, the esophagus, stomach, duodenum, and from below, the colon and terminal ileum, have proved relatively straightforward to intubate, by pushing flexible tubes with particular characteristics.

The tips of the endoscopes used for these purposes have variable radius curvature to adapt to bends in the GI tract, torsional stiffness and resistance to excessive lateral deviation from the axis of the introducing force. Thus, these endoscopes are steerable during forward advancement in relation to fixed internal structures. In upper endoscopy these fixed structures include the entire esophagus and the second, third and fourth parts of the duodenum. In the colon the fixed structures are the rectum, the descending colon, the ascending colon, and cecum. When the relatively mobile portions of these organs are traversed by an endoscope, the distendable and free-moving parts, such as sigmoid colon, transverse colon and the gastric body, can be kept relatively straight between fixed bowel at either end. The fixity of these structures allows further advance of the endoscope without carrying the gut forward by means of friction with the intestinal wall.

The small intestine (from the ligament of Treitz) to the cecum is, however, unfixed except by its mesenteric attachment. This allows the intestine a great freedom of movement in almost all directions. Attempting to push a flexible tube into such an unsupported structure is inclined to be met with limited success. This is because the small bowel has a very great capacity to elongate (around 3 m of normal length, stretching to an extreme of 6 m when measured at necropsy). Further to this, the friction between the intubation tube and the intestine is greater than the friction between the intestine and its surrounding structures. The tube therefore tends, firstly, to elongate the intestine when pushed and, secondly, tends to move the intestine with which it is in contact in relation to surrounding bowel loops.

These problems will always beset intubation of the small intestine using an axial advancing pressure. The further problem in the small intestine is that at both top and bottom, the entrance to the intestine is an inconveniently long way from either the mouth or the anus.

An alternative method of intubation for the purposes of endoscope examination of the small intestine is to arrange for the endoscope to be pulled rather than pushed to the length of the organ.

Pulling the enteroscope through the small intestine with a previously inserted guidewire ("rope-way" enteroscopy) is painful, requires general anesthesia and has not achieved widespread application.

through the pylorus into the duodenum. Brief insufflations further assist it round the duodenal loop. This procedure is at least as quick as the "piggy-back" method (2-3 min) and is more comfortable for the patient. In around 10% of cases it is not possible to push the sonde enteroscope through the pylorus; then the "piggy-back" method is employed (personal observations).

Fluroscopic passive

The sonde endoscope is passed into the gastric antrum, the balloon inflated and then it is left to be propelled by gastroduodenal peristalsis. This is the most comfortable of the three techniques but may add 1/2 to 1 h to the whole procedure.

Other sonde enteroscopes

Other long enteroscopes have been used ES1-2000, (Pentax) and VSB 2000 and SSIF V1 KAI (Olympus). The latter showed a significant advance in that an instrument channel allows the mucosa to be pushed away from the otherwise passive endoscope tip, and the amount of mucosa examined was increased. The former has video technology, and a deflectable tip is added to the later VSB model. The main disadvantage these instruments have in common is their great diameter, preventing perinasal passage in very many patients.

Progress through the small intestine

After the enteroscope reaches the ligament of Treitz, the balloon is left inflated to around 2 cm in diameter, and onward progress may be encouraged with the use of a prokinetic agent. However, when this was formally studied, no benefit was observed The patient relaxes in bed and, in some cases, may receive further sedation to assist sleep during the ensuing hours. The attendant, usually a specialist gastrointestinal nurse, then introduces 20-30 cm of the enteroscope every half to 1 h for the ensuing 6-8 h. The rate of insertion of the tube is matched to onward progress of the balloon using X-ray guidance every 1-2 h. The skilled attendant is generally able to tell if there is gastric looping because of resistance to insertion of the tube.

Any gastric looping is undone during X-ray screening. Eight to ten hours are usually allotted for allowing the tube to pass into the distal small intestine. This fits in with the normal working day, although extra time may be allotted for those patients with a particular requirement to get to the distal ileum. The procedure can be extended by 3-4 h or, in rare cases, the enteroscope may be left in place overnight. In the latter case, the patient needs to be supervised by a specialized gastrointestinal nurse familiar with the equipment and the procedure.

In some cases very little progress is made due to apparent lack of peristalsis in the small intestine. It has become apparent that the main cause for this slow progress in the small intestine is prior ingestion of opioid analgesia. Even a relatively mild preparation such as Dextropropoxyphene (usually taken in combination with Paracetamol) may cause major small intestinal stasis. This problem became apparent during the investigation of patients with rheumatoid arthritis who take analgesics on most days.

The enteroscopic examination

The views obtained during sonde enteroscopy are limited by an inability to actively deflect the tip, as would normally be the case with other gastrointestinal endoscopes. This constraint arises by sacrificing tip-deflecting wires in favor of achieving a narrow and very flexible scope, which therefore is more likely to penetrate deep into the small intestine.

Water or air insufflation?

When the instrument is deemed to have travelled sufficiently far, examination may commence and all the views are obtained during withdrawal of the instrument. The view is obtained by the insufflation of either air or water. The advantage of water-insufflation over air-insufflation is that water may be infused continuously throughout the withdrawal phase when the patient is being examined, whereas air

Sonde enteroscopy

The most successful technique for achieving extensive examination of the small intestine is the use of a traction balloon on the tip of the endoscope. This instrument is called the sonde enteroscope. This endoscope traverses the length of the small intestine by means of small intestinal contractions. An inflated balloon of sufficient size (2-3 cm in diameter) is used to distend the small intestine. This distention force provokes peristalsis-like activity which, over the course of some hours, propels the balloon, together with the attached endoscope, down into the distal intestine.

There are a number of drawbacks with sonde enteroscopy, some of these drawbacks inherent in the technique, while others may in the future be overcome with advances in technology. There is, however, one overriding advantage with the sonde technique – its ability to examine the entire small intestine. Push-enteroscopy is limited to the proximal 100 cm or so of small intestine.

Instrumentation and technique

Much of the report at work has been done with the 2.7 m in length and 5 mm diameter sonde enteroscope (Olympus SIF-SW). This instrument is long enough to reach the cecum, flexible enough to traverse multiple small bowel, multiple small intestinal loops, and narrow enough to minimize friction with the mucosa and to allow passage through the nose. The distal tip has a 4 cm latex sleeve, the distal end bound tightly to the scope tip and the proximal to the endoscope 4 cm higher up. An air channel has its exit under the sleeve, allowing it to be inflated to form a near-spherical balloon surrounding the endoscope tip. This balloon, when in use, can vary between 5 mm and 3 cm in diameter according to requirements. A further channel through the endoscope can be used to introduce water or air at the intestinal lumen. Fiberoptic bundles deliver illumination to the tip and carry the image from a wide-angled lens (120°) at the tip, to a standard endoscopy eyepiece. Images are usually captured by a video camera attached to the eyepiece. There are no facilities for either biopsy or for the introduction of a catheter to deliver energy for therapeutic purposes.

Introducing the sonde endoscope into the small intestine

In almost all cases, the sonde endoscope is passed transnasally. Some workers have used the oral route but this limits the ability of the patient to keep the tube down for hours at a time. The diameter of the endoscope is similar to nasogastric aspiration tubes, used for continuous gastric decompression in patients with acute abdominal conditions. The ability to tolerate such a tube for many hours has therefore been well tried and tested.

The diameter of the endoscope is such as to pass very neatly through the nasal cavity in all but a tiny minority of patients (1.5%).

Intravenous sedation and topical nasal and pharyngeal anesthesia precede the introduction of the endoscope. There are three techniques for introducing the instrument into the small intestine: (1) "piggy-back," (2) fluroscopic/active, and (3) fluroscopic/passive.

"Piggy-back" enteroscopy
This was first described by Lewis and others in 1987. The sonde enteroscope is passed transnasally into the distal stomach. A second upper gastrointestinal endoscope (or enteroscope, or colonoscope) is passed perorally into the stomach. The sonde enteroscope is identified and a suture at its distal tip is grasped with biopsy forceps and passed through the second endoscope. In the original description, both endoscopes are then advanced into the distal duodenum. The sonde enteroscope is then released, the balloon inflated and the introducing endoscope withdrawn.

Fluroscopic/active
In most cases, however, the sonde enteroscope can be pushed to the ligament of Treitz simply using X-ray guidance, without the use of a second endoscope. In this case, the balloon is used to assist introduction by brief insufflations, to centralize in the antrum. Then it can be pushed

can only be injected intermittently. Continuous air-insufflation during the 20-30 min of examination would lead to unacceptable small intestinal distention and discomfort. The further advantage of water-insufflation is that fine mucosal detail can be observed, intestinal villi being individually visible, suspended in the water and without unwanted light reflection. Active bleeding may sometimes be traced to a "plume" of hemorrhage into the clear water rather than as a diffuse layer of fresh blood extending proximally and distally on the mucosa with air insufflation.

Abdominal palpation and "mucosal pushing"

Although the endoscope tip cannot be moved by controls, abdominal palpation enables the intestine to be moved with respect to the tip and, in most patients, this contributes significantly to the amount of mucosa that can be seen. The mucosa can be pushed away from the tip with one prototype instrument that is equipped with an instrument channel (Olympus SSIF-V11 KA1), but this instrument is usually restricted to the relatively unsatisfactory oral route of intubation.

Controlling the rate of withdrawl

As the enteroscope is withdrawn, the more proximal part of the tube moves more readily in relation to the intestine and the distal part of the tube. This effect is due to summative friction. The result of this is that the intestine comes together in pleats, concertinalike, proximal to the distal tip. This effect can be minimized by abdominal palpation, encouraging an even and controlled exit of the endoscope. Nevertheless, the sudden release of the segment of pleating may lead to a rush of intestine, past the endoscope tip, perhaps 10-15 cm at a time. This leads to the intestine moving too fast for satisfactory examination. One solution to this problem is the rapid insufflation of the balloon to stop the movement of the intestine. This may be done by the means of a 30 ml syringe containing air. An alternative is to use a sphygmomanometer insufflation bulb in closed circuit with the balloon.

This bulb is placed on the floor and compressed by the foot-"foot brake," enabling the hands of the operator to be kept free for withdrawal and abdominal palpitation (personal observations).

Smooth muscle relaxant drugs

The temporary reduction of intestinal contractility after the injection of hyoscine or glucagon can facilitate enteroscopic views. Constant movement of the intestine sometimes can impair adequate examination. However, the duration of action of intravenously administered hyoscine may be very brief, less than 5 min, and repeated dosing will be required to maintain the intestine in a state of relaxation for the 20 min of the examination.

This is not a problem during therapeutic endoscopy using a push enteroscope because of the briefer nature of that form of examination.

If hyoscine is not used, it is possible to limit the loss of views engendered by the endoscope moving back too quickly and too far. When this rapid withdrawal occurs, the balloon is inflated to fullness, the withdrawing action is reversed rapidly, and 20-30 cm of endoscope is reinserted. This maneuver often results in a distension-induced prokinetic contraction, and a few centimetres of lost ground can be regained. This, of course, relies upon the fact that contraction is not hindered by the use of the smooth-muscle relaxant. Using the above techniques, it is estimated that between 50% and 70% of the mucosal area is examined. This may improve to 75% using the mucosal "push-away" technique.

How much small intestine distal to the final insertion point remains unexamined?

Before the examination commences, the gastric loop is withdrawn under X-ray control, until the enteroscope can be seen to be foreshortening the lesser curve of the stomach. The depth of insertion into the small intestine is then estimated by subtracting the nasopyloric distance, usually estimated at 60 cm, with the lesser curves straightened out. The length of enteroscope in the small intestine is then subtracted from a notional 3 m length of small bowel. This gives the length of intestine unexamined. The method is relatively crude because of the unknown amount of pleating over the endoscope tip. Further assistance in this can be achieved by the injection of an iodine-based radio-opaque contrast material through the enteroscope and its passage followed to the cecum using X-ray imaging. This can have the additional bonus of revealing anatomical abnormalities in the unexamined portion of ileum.

Indications for and limitations of sonde enteroscopy

In most cases with the need for enteroscopy, the push-enteroscopy is the procedure of first choice. It is much quicker, the intestine intubated may be examined more carefully, under more direct control and it has the ability to perform multiple biopsies and deliver therapy to tougher lesions such as arterovenous malformations.

Indications
If, however, lesions are suspected further than 100 cm beyond to the ligament of Treitz, the capacity for sonde enteroscopy to read deeper is needed. The following are its usual indications:
- Occult G.I bleeding and negative push-enteroscopy
- ? Crohn's disease in the ileum
- ? Meckel's diverticulum
- ? Extent of precancerous lesions

Limitations
- No biopsies or therapeutic facilities
- Partial views of lumen
- Poorly controlled brief views of mucosa
- Prolonged intubation
- Normal peristalsis required

Complications
Two perforations have been reported, not from the same center, using the Olympus SS1F-SW. One case was related to operator error in which water was infused in excess into the balloon, and the other was apparently caused by the balloon disturbing a pre-existing jejunal ulcer. Both patients made an uneventful recovery after appropriate surgical intervention (personal observations).

Other complications have been mild: abdominal pain during the procedure; epistaxis, self-terminating, occurs in 6.5% of patients.

Suggested reading

Gostout CJ (1996) Sonde-enteroscopy: technical depth of inserts and yield of lesions. Gastrointest Endosc Clin NAM 6:777-847

Lewis BS, Waye JD (1987) Total small bowel enteroscopy. Gastrointest Endosc 33:435-438

Morris AJ, Wasson LA, MacKenzie JF (1992) Small bowel enteroscopy in un-diagnosed gastro-intestinal blood loss. Gut 33:887-889

Sonde enteroscopy

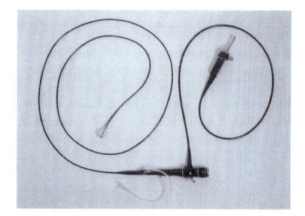

Fig. 1. Sonde enteroscope

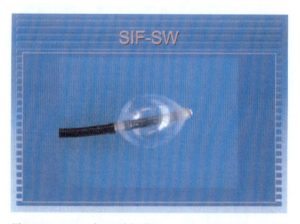

Fig 2. A near spherical balloon surrounding the endoscope tip

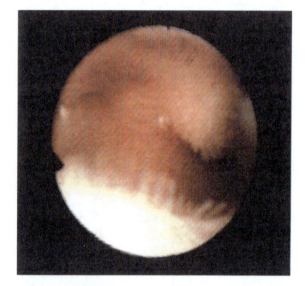

Fig. 3. Normal villi

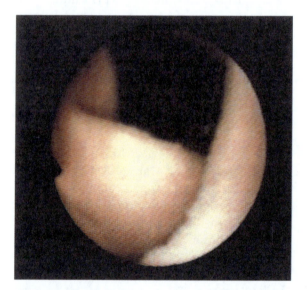

Fig. 4. Partial villous atrophy in NSAID enteropathy

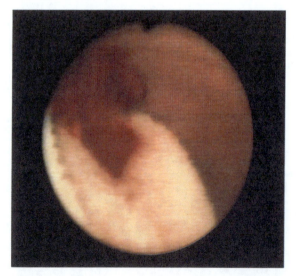

Fig. 5. Water insufflation localizes the source of hemorrage in small bowel

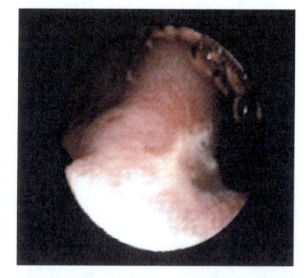

Fig. 6. Meckel's diverticulum with ulceration of adjacent ileum (underwater view)

Push enteroscopy

G. Gay, M. Pennazio, J.S. Delmotte, F.P. Rossini

Standard push enteroscopy

Push enteroscopy is a technique in which a long flexible endoscope is passed orally, allowing exploration of the small bowel beyond the anatomic limit reachable by conventional esophagogastroduodenoscopy.

Standard or thin-caliber colonoscopes have been employed for exploration of the proximal jejunum.

Recent years have seen the development of both optical fiber and video flexible enteroscopes, specially designed to study the small bowel (Table 1).

They are provided with guidewires that provide good mobility of the tip even when the instrument is inserted deep within the small bowel. The wide field of view allows optimal vision with good image definition. Through the biopsy channel, 2.8 mm in diameter, not only targeted biopsies but also subsidiary operative techniques may be performed.

Push enteroscopy is a method of short duration (20-30 min, plus time needed for any subsidiary techniques) and in general it is well tolerated, provided it is performed under adequate sedation if the patient is conscious; more frequently, the investigation is carried out in a surgical unit, with the anesthetized patient under respiratory assistance.

To avoid looping in the stomach, an overtube is backloaded onto the instrument before the examination is begun. This has the function of stiffening the enteroscope so that the push can transit successfully along its entire length. Before introducing either the overtube or the enteroscope they must be abundantly lubricated.

Table 1. Video push-type enteroscopes

	OLYMPUS			PENTAX	FUJINON
Model	SIF 200	SIF 100	XSIF-Q140	VSB-2900	EN7-MR2
Field of view	140°	140°	120°	100°	120°
Depth of field	5-100 mm	5-100 mm	3-100 mm	5-100 mm	5-100 mm
Outer diam. of insertion tube	11.2 mm	11.3 mm	10.5 mm	9.8 mm	11.5 mm
Range of tip bending:					
• Up-down	180°	180°	180°	130°	180°
• Right-left	160°	160°	160°	130°	160°
Inner diameter of biopsy channel	2.8 mm	2.8 mm	2.8 mm	2.8 mm	2.8 mm
Working length	2,000 mm	2,175 mm	2,675 mm	2,500 mm	2,000 mm
Overall length		2,475 mm	2,975 mm	2,820 mm	2,340 mm

With the patient in left lateral decubitus, the enteroscope is introduced orally into the gastric cavity, taking care not to distend the stomach with excessive insufflation; it is then pushed into the third section of the duodenum. The enteroscope is retracted to straighten it, and the overtube inserted along the enteroscope, kept taut to avoid looping, until its distal tip reaches the second section of the duodenum. Further progress of the endoscope within the small bowel is facilitated by changes of decubitus, manual pressure on the abdomen, and hooking and retraction movements.

Fluoroscopy is useful but not indispensible to position the overtube; the correct position is confirmed by the retrogade flow of bile leaking from the valve situated at the proximal tip of the overtube, with the enteroscope under suction.

The use of drugs to reduce gut motility, such as anticholinergic drugs, glucagon, or topical ottilonium bromide, may facilitate insertion and optimize endoscopic vision. During both insertion and retraction phases, the entire mucosal surface of the lumen may be accurately evaluated. If an area is not clearly identified, the enteroscope may be reintroduced to achieve more precise visualization.

Videorecording of the examination is of great help: since the session may be reviewed on the screen, it is possible to evaluate some images that, due to the rapid movement of the loops, escaped examination during retraction of the instrument.

The incidence of complications in this method is low, comparable to that of esophagogastroduodenoscopy. Complications reported in the literature are: trauma to the esophagogastric mucosa; very rare duodenojejunal perforations; Mallory-Weiss tear; acute pancreatitis; acute facial swelling caused by the enlargement of the parotid and submaxillary salivary glands. All these complications are generally caused by the use of the overtube.

The new overtubes, with differentiated rigidity, distal and proximal tips in Goretex, and a more rounded distal tip, are easier to use and reduce the risk of complications.

The depth of insertion of the instrument may be verified radiographically or with fluoroscopy; however, note that the technique does not allow the depth to be determined with absolute certainty, owing to the variable telescoping of the bowel on the instrument.

At present, the limit of push enteroscopy is that it does not permit exploration of the entire small bowel; the entire jejunum can be visualized, but only occasionally the first loops of the ileum.

The push enteroscopy main indications are:
- Obscure gastrointestinal bleeding
- Unexplained diarrhea and malabsorption
- Small bowel neoplasias
- Surveillance of precancerous lesions: Peutz-Jeghers syndrome, familial adenomatous and familial juvenile polyposis, human non-polyposis colorectal cancer syndrome, celiac disease, Crohn's disease
- Further endoscopic exploration and tissue diagnosis of radiographically suspected disease
- To perform therapeutic procedures

Double-way enteroscopy

In order to visualize the totality of the small bowel mucosa, the use of a push enteroscope introduced anally has recently been suggested. Depending on the patient's level of tolerance, double-way enteroscopy may be carried out during the same session or on successive days. The lower procedure is more difficult than the upper one because of the flexibility of the enteroscope; it is thus necessary to use a special overtube. However, even using the overtube, insertion of the push enteroscope into the ileum is difficult and time-consuming. In favorable circumstances (10% of cases) with the double-way technique it is possible to explore the totality of the small bowel. To confirm the totality of intubation, a bleeding biopsy is performed during the upper exploration and must be seen during the lower exploration.

Special indications for push enteroscopy

Access to the common bile duct after Roux-en-Y gastrojejunostomy

Push enteroscopy may be useful for the exploration of loops of the jejunal limb after gastric surgery, or to access the common bile or pancreatic duct to carry out a cholangiogram in patients with Roux-en-Y gastrojejunostomy.

Placement of percutaneous jejunostomies

For long-term enteral feeding into the jejunum, the technique of direct percutaneous jejunostomy (PEJ) is more satisfactory than passing a feeding tube through a percutaneous endoscopic gastrostomy (PEG). The best indication for this procedure is in patients who are at risk for aspiration, or in cases of gastric outlet or duodenal obstruction. The jejunal loop must be located close enough to the abdominal wall to allow transillumination; it is essential to proceed quickly after its identification in order to avoid the disappearance of the transilluminated area.

A novel technique for the insertion of a jejunal feeding tube using an enteroscope and a laparoscope has recently been described. A jejunostomy tube is positioned using direct puncture of a jejunal loop at enteroscopy. Under laparascopic control, the needle is passed through the anterior abdominal wall.

Enteroscopy-Enteroclysis

Double-contrast enteroclysis of the small bowel is a radiological method in which the contrast medium is administered directly into the proximal portion of the small bowel via a probe introduced nasally or orally. In general the procedure is uncomfortable for the patient, and correct positioning of the probe is sometimes difficult even if it is done under fluoroscopic guidance.

A combined method has been proposed, which involves performing a push enteroscopy followed, in the same session, by enteroclysis in cases where the endoscopic examinition is negative. Enteroclysis is facilitated by positioning a guidewire in the proximal jejunum during enteroscopy. The guidewire is left in place when the enteroscope is removed; the probe to inject contrast medium is pushed along this until it reaches the inferior limit explored endoscopically.

Endoscopic appearance of the normal small bowel mucosa

It is not easy to distinguish the jejunum from the ileum, because there is no sharp demarcation. However, it is useful to keep in mind that the jejunum is thicker and its lumen is wider: 25-30 mm of diameter on moderate insufflation. In the same conditions, the diameter of the ileum is 15-25 mm.

The mucosa of the jejunum is different from the mucosa of the ileum: in the jejunum we can see the transverse folds of Kerckring; valvulae conniventes are as regularly spaced and as sharp as in the duodenum; they are numerous, thick and high and do not disappear on insufflation.

The height of these folds in the jejunum is about 2-5 mm; in the ileum they are progressively fewer and less prominent, and transverse folds encircle the lumen but only for two-thirds of the circumference. The height of a fold is 0.5-3 mm in this intestinal segment.

The submucosal vascular network is not evident in the jejunum, while it is visible in the last ileal loops.

In young people, the last loops of the ileum present a fairly regular nodular aspect (1-2 mm of diameter); these are the lymphoid islets.

Chromoscopy

Detailed observation of the musosa can be achieved by injecting a 0.05 % solution of indigo carmine through the biopsy channel with a Teflon catheter.

Under-water view

In this technique, the physical properties of water are exploited. By filling the lumen with water – 50-200 ml – after suction of excess air, it is possible to observe minute mucosal details.

Suggested reading

Chong J, Tagle M, Barkin JS, Reimer DK (1995) Small bowel push fiberoptic enteroscopy for patients with occult gastrointestinal bleeding or suspected small bowel pathology. Am J Gastroenterol 89:2142-2146

Gay G, Delmotte JS (1996) Modalités techniques de l'entéroscopie sonde et de l'entéroscopie poussée par simple et double voie. Acta Endosc 26:239-247

Pennazio M, Arrigoni A, Risio M, Spandre M, Rossini FP (1995) Clinical evaluation of push type enteroscopy. Endoscopy 27:164-170

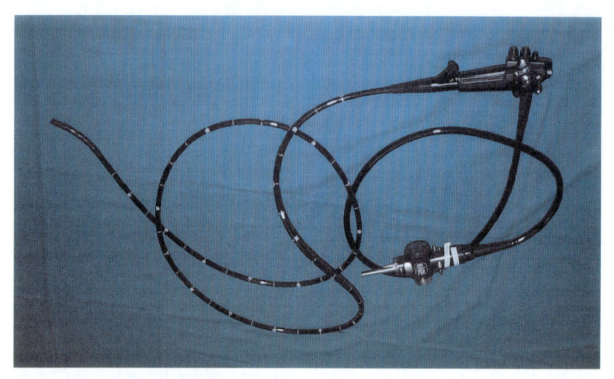

Fig. 1. Push enteroscope (Olympus XSIF-Q140)

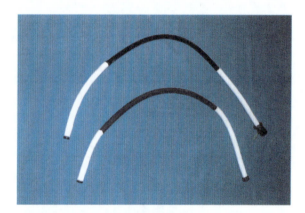

Fig. 2. Overtubes for push enteroscopy

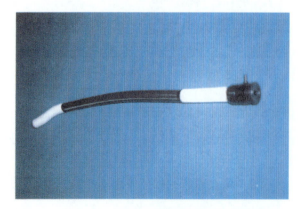

Fig. 3. Special overtube for double-way enteroscopy

Atlas of Enteroscopy

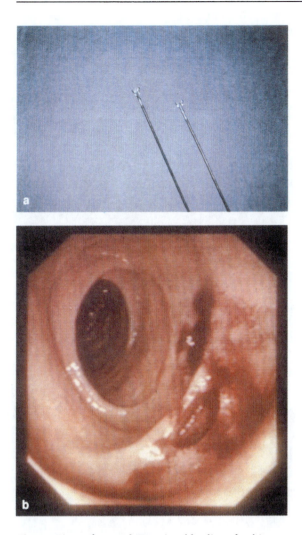

Fig. 4. a Biopsy forceps. b Transient bleeding after biopsy: "open fish-mouth appearance"

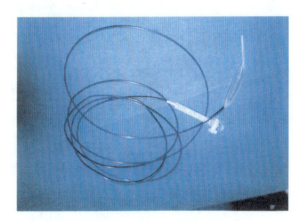

Fig. 5. Balloon dilator

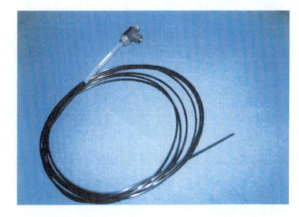

Fig. 6. Heather probe

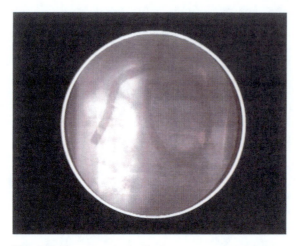
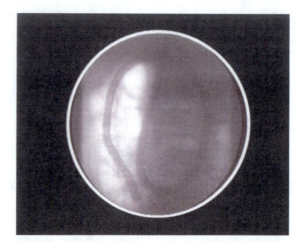

Figs. 7, 8. Fluoroscopic check: the enteroscope is inserted in the jejunum

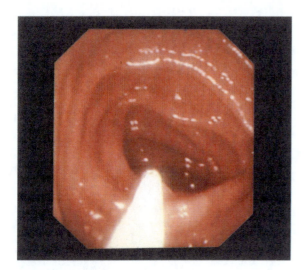

Fig. 9. Teflon catheter collecting jejunal juice

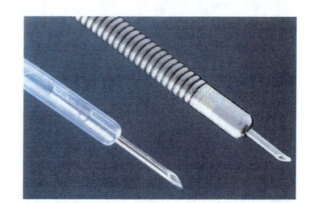

Fig. 10. Injection needles

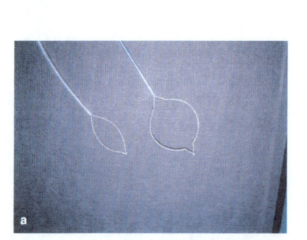
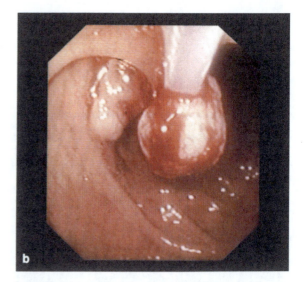

Fig. 11. a Polypectomy snares of different sizes. **b** Endoscopic polypectomy

Atlas of Enteroscopy

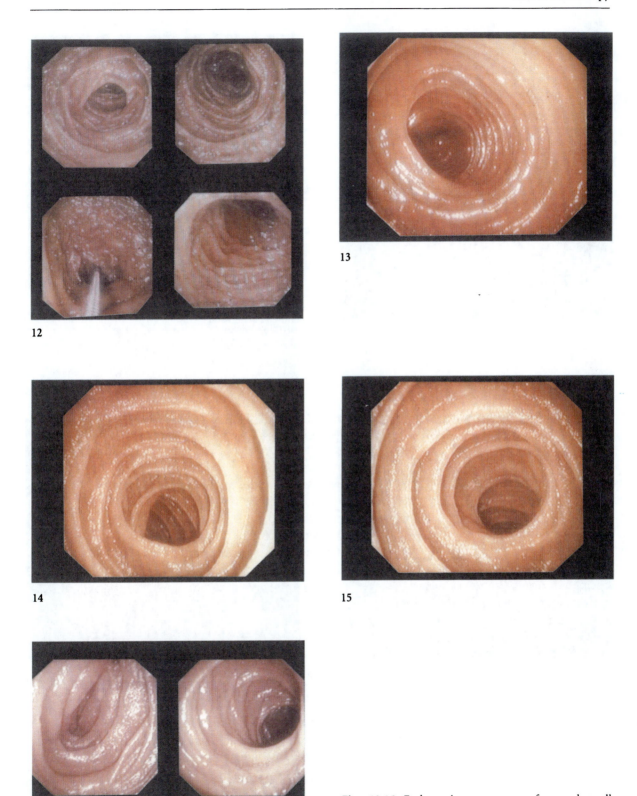

12

13

14

15

16

Figs. 12-16. Endoscopic appearances of normal small bowel mucosa

49

Push enteroscopy

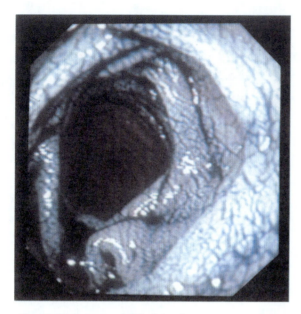

Fig. 17. Chromoscopy of the jejunal mucosa

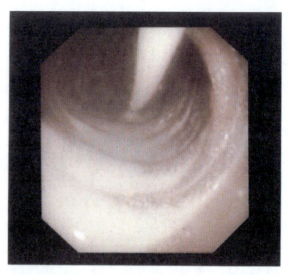

Fig. 18. Sectorial perendoscopic contrastography with diluted barium sulfate

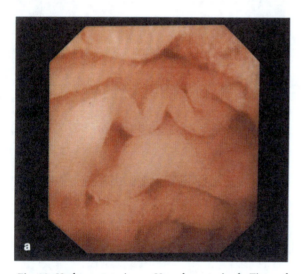
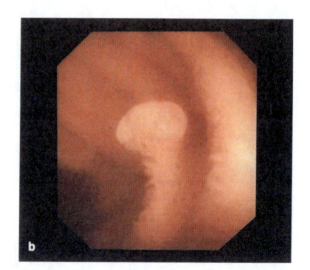

Fig. 19. *Under-water view.* a Vascular ectasias b Tiny polyp

Intraoperative enteroscopy

G. Gay, M. Pennazio, J.S. Delmotte, F.P. Rossini

Intraoperative enteroscopy is an accurate method for examination of the entire small bowel. It may be carried out with a standard or thin-caliber colonoscope or with a push or sonde enteroscope. The advent of the modern push videoenteroscopes has brought about considerable improvement in terms of reducing trauma to the mucosa, improving endoscopic vision, reaching more distal segments of the small bowel, as well as making all therapeutic procedures possible. Exploration of the small bowel by both direct vision and palpation, or only laparoscopically, should be accomplished before the scope is introduced into the small bowel. This procedure can diagnose tumors, large vascular lesions, and Meckel's diverticulum. The finding of such lesions will obviate the need for intraoperative enteroscopy. The endoscope is mainly inserted orally and by enterotomy. The risk of infection using the latter way can be prevented by coating the endoscope with sterile light tissue. If a push enteroscope is available, it is passed orally and advanced up to the duodenojejunal flexure, with the aid of an overtube previously backloaded onto the enteroscope and positioned, after insertion of the enteroscope, in the second portion of the duodenum. Intubation of the duodenum is easier if it is done before the abdomen is opened. A non-crushing clamp should be placed on the ileocecal junction to prevent colonic distension. If intra-abdominal adhesions are encountered, they should be lysed to facilitate progression of the enteroscope. The surgeon then grasps the tip of the scope and holds a short segment of small bowel for endoscopic inspection. The mucosa should be examined mainly during insertion because on withdrawal, mucosal trauma are difficult to distinguish from vascular malformations. While the endoscopist observes the mucosa, the surgeon examines the serosal surface by transillumination. The mucosa of the small bowel is best visualized by setting a clamp every 30 cm of examination of the small bowel. Rather than using a clamp, an assistant can manually clamp the short segments of the small bowel; this will result in less mucosal trauma. In order to examine the entire small bowel, the surgeon telescopes the small bowel onto the enteroscope and facilitates progress of the instrument with external counterpressure or by reducing loops in the stomach – if an overtube is not used – and in the small bowel. After segmental inspection, the bowel is evacuated of air and the same method is applied for the next 30 cm. Identified lesions are marked serosally or treated endoscopically. Moreover, videomonitoring allows the endoscopist and surgeon to work in close cooperation. Every movement needs to be made cautiously: minimal inflation, progression under visual control, frequent looks at the mesentery in order to avoid excessive stretching.

The endoscopic procedure usually takes 30-45 min. The diagnostic yield of intraoperative enteroscopy has ranged from 70% to 100% (Tables 1, 2).

Intraoperative enteroscopy is a difficult, time-consuming technique that is often traumatic to the bowel; thus, the decision to perform it requires a careful balancing of the risks and benefits of the procedure. The success of the technique is directly correlated both to a careful preoperative evaluation of the strategy to be adopted and to close cooperation between the surgeon and the endoscopist during the examination.

Table 1. Intraoperative enteroscopy: indications

- Chronic transfusion-dependent gastrointestinal bleeding, the source of which has not been identified by previous radiologic and endoscopic examinations
- In cases of torrential bleeding thought to be of small bowel origin when the need for emergency surgery precludes a complete preoperative work-up
- To localize the precise site of lesions found on sonde enteroscopy
- To guide selection of the appropriate extent of gut resection
- Peutz-Jeghers syndrome, familial adenomatous and familial juvenile polyposis

Table 2. Intraoperative enteroscopy: complications

- Mucosal lacerations
- Submucosal hematoma
- Small bowel ischemia
- Small bowel perforation
- Prolonged postoperative ileus
- Wound infection
- Postoperative death

Suggested reading

Cave DR, Cooley JS (1996) Intraoperative enteroscopy: indications and techniques. Gastrointest Endosc Clin N Am 6:793-802

Lewis BS, Jeffrey MD, Wengers S, Waye JD (1991) Small bowel enteroscopy and intraoperative enteroscopy for obscure gastrointestinal bleeding. Am J Gastroenterol 86:171-174

Mathus-Vliegen EMH, Tytgat GNJ (1986) Intraoperative endoscopy: technique, indications and results. Gastrointest Endosc 32:381-384

Atlas of Enteroscopy

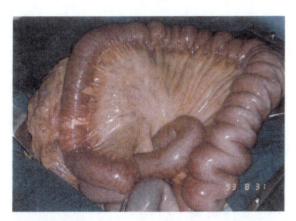

Fig. 1. Intraoperative enteroscopy: the instrument is inserted up to the ileocecal junction

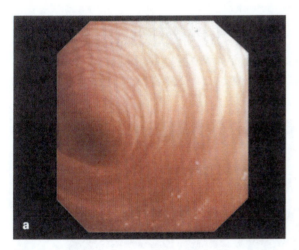
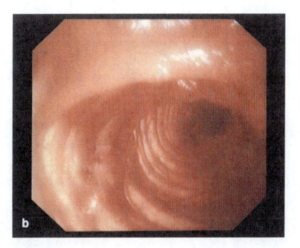

Fig. 2. a, b Endoscopic view of the intestinal lumen during intraoperative enteroscopy

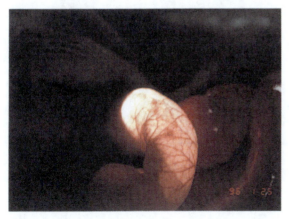

Fig. 3. View of the vascular network by transillumination of the small bowel

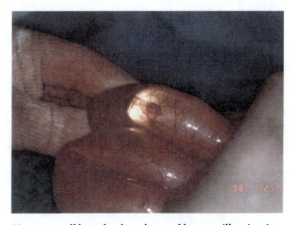

Fig. 4. A small bowel polyp observed by transillumination

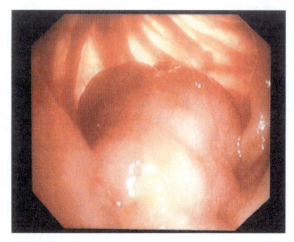

Fig. 5. A big ileal polyp

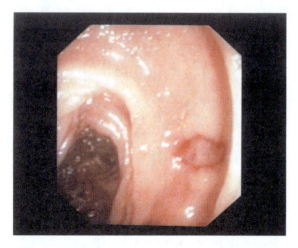

Fig. 6. Mucosal laceration during intraoperative enteroscopy

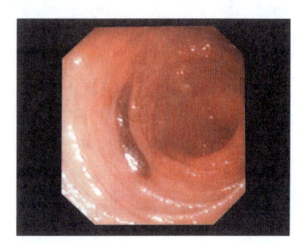

Fig. 7. Submucosal hematoma

Laparoscopically assisted enteroscopy

P. Bauret, J.M. Fabre

Technique

The investigation is realized in a surgical unit on an anesthetized patient under respiratory assitance. An exploratory laparoscopy is first performed, and the small bowel is examined using two atraumatic grasping forceps from the ileocecal valve to the ligament of Treitz (Figs. 1, 2).

A video push-type enteroscope (Olympus SIF 100) and its overtube (to avoid gastric loop of the endoscope) with a working length of 210 cm are then introduced per os and inserted beyond the duodenojejunal flexure.

Progression of the endoscope tip toward the ileum is possible by combining the push of the enteroscope by the endoscopist and the bowel telescoping on to the scope by the surgeon using laparoscopic forceps (Figs. 3, 4).

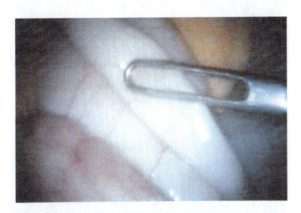

Fig. 1. Laparoscopic small bowel exploration

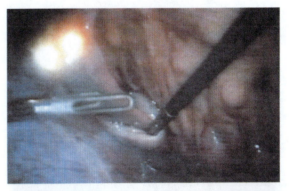

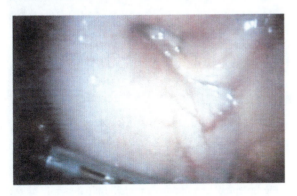

Fig. 2. Ileal melanoma discovered at laparoscopy

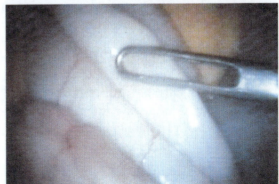

Figs. 3 (*top*) and **4** (*bottom*). Bowel telescoping on the scope

The lumen and external surface of the transilluminated intestine are inspected by the endoscopist and the surgeon in 10 cm segments (Fig. 5).

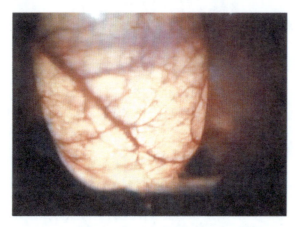

Fig. 5. Transilluminated intestine by enteroscope light

Examination is only performed during intubation since mucosal trauma may occur with the small bowel pleating, causing artifacts. When an abnormality is identified, a small serosal suture is placed to mark the site.

Laparoscopically assisted enteroscopy per os without enterotomy allows mucosa and serosa examination of the entire jejunum and, in some cases, of the proximal ileum and could avoid unnecessary laparotomies.

Indications

• Investigation of small bowel X-ray abnormalities located in the mid-small bowel or in the proximal ileum rarely reached by push enteroscopy (Figs. 6, 7).

• Exploration of obscure gastrointestinal bleeding with negative previous evaluation by oesophagogastroduodenoscopy, colonoscopy and push enteroscopy, especially in patients under 50 years if a small bowel tumor or a Meckel's diverticulum is suspected.

• Evaluation of disease extension, particularly in cases of vascular abnormalities (Fig. 8).

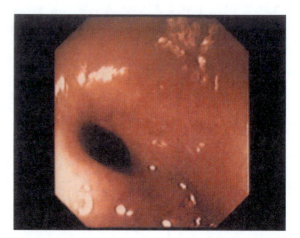

Fig. 6. Post-NSAID small bowel stenosis

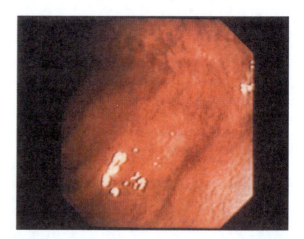

Fig. 7. Ileal short mucosal ischemia due to a microscopic carcinoid

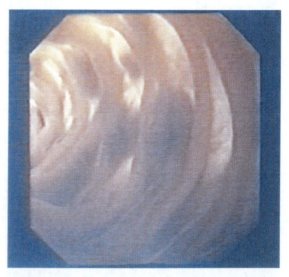

Fig. 8. Jejunal angiomatosis transilluminated only by the laparoscopic light

Contraindications

- Specific contraindication for the pneumoperitoneum
- Cardiac or respiratory insufficiency
- Diffuse intra-abdominal adhesions from previous laparotomies
- Large abdominal wall hernia

Complications

The complications are mainly mucosal trauma and serosal tearing. Anterograde inspection circumvents the problem of differentiating trauma from subtle mucosal abnormalities. In one personal experience no severe complications (perforation, prolonged ileus, infection) have been observed (Fig. 9).

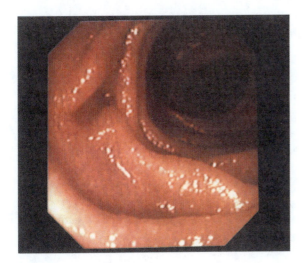

Fig. 9. Mucosal trauma

GASTROINTESTINAL BLEEDING

Emergency bleeding

Management of obscure gastrointestinal bleeding

Angiodysplasias

NSAID enteropathy

Meckel's diverticulum – Jejunoileal diverticulosis

Emergency bleeding

G. Gay, F.P. Rossini, J.S. Delmotte, M. Pennazio

Small bowel bleeding accounts for 25% to 30% of acute lower gastrointestinal bleeding and represents 5% of upper and lower gastrointestinal hemorrhages. The first priority in this situation is the restoration of cardiovascular stability. After this step and only after, the etiology and the therapy of bleeding can be considered. Under these conditions, the diagnosis and therapy for emergency bleeding cannot be well standardized because of the difference in availability of certain techniques, as well as the experience and training of the physician.

Clinical presentation

Upper gastrointestinal bleeding. In this situation, the approach after adequate resuscitation should be: esophagogastroduodenoscopy and, if the papilla of Vater has not been adequately visualized, a lateral duodenoscope should be employed in order to exclude a wirsungorragia. Push enteroscopy should be considered in selected cases (persistent bleeding and no sources found by previous examinations).

The clinical situation is more complex in acute lower gastrointestinal bleeding; from a practical point of view, it is possible to distinguish different clinical presentations.

Massive lower hemorrhage: the following algorithm should be followed.

Massive lower hemorrhage
↓
Angiography
↓
Intraoperative endoscopy (colonoscopy, enteroscopy)

Severe acute lower gastrointestinal bleeding, which can be divided into:

Severe permanent bleeding (20% of cases)

```
┌─────────────────────────────────────┐
│ 1 - Bedside proctoscopy             │
│ 2 - Rule out upper GI source (10%)  │
│     no source found                 │
└─────────────────────────────────────┘
```

```
┌─────────────────────────────────────┐
│ 3 - Angiography (>1 cc/min)         │
└─────────────────────────────────────┘
```

(−)
```
┌─────────────────────────────────────┐
│ 4 - Emergency colonoscopy           │
└─────────────────────────────────────┘
```

(−)
```
┌─────────────────────────────────────┐
│ 5 - Push enteroscopy                │
└─────────────────────────────────────┘
```

(−)
```
┌─────────────────────────────────────┐
│ 6 - Surgical exploration            │
└─────────────────────────────────────┘
```

Intermittent severe lower gastrointestinal bleeding (80% of cases). In this situation, bleeding usually is self-limiting. It is possible in relation with the clinical context, the available equipment and the experience of the team to choose the best diagnostic procedure in order to find the source of bleeding (see chapter "Management of obscure gastrointestinal bleeding").

Suggested reading

Lewis B (1994) Small intestinal bleeding. In: Gastrointestinal bleeding II. Freedman LS (ed) Gastroenterol Clin North Am 23:67-91

Shapiro MJ (1994) The role of the radiologist in the management of gastrointestinal bleeding. In: Gastrointestinal Bleeding II. Freedman LS (ed) Gastroenterol. Clin North Am 93:123-181

Management of obscure gastrointestinal bleeding

M. Pennazio, F.P. Rossini

Obscure gastrointestinal bleeding (OGIB) is most commonly defined as acute or chronic blood loss, intermittent or continuous, with iron-deficiency anemia and heme-positive stool. The source of bleeding is still undetected in 3% to 5% of patients even after thorough upper and lower endoscopy. Bleeding is more likely to continue in these patients, and the site of bleeding may be in the small bowel or, less frequently, the biliary tree or the pancreas. In the small bowel, the most frequent cause of bleeding (70-80%) is secondary to single, sporadic or, more rarely, diffuse angiodysplasias. The second-most-common source is primitive or metastatic neoplasias (Table 1).

Unless bleeding is massive, the cause is often difficult to diagnose if it is located within the small bowel. The small bowel's length and tortuosity makes it less accessible than the stomach and colon, thus limiting the diagnostic accuracy of conventional procedures.

The most important diagnostic procedures used to evaluate patients with OGIB are: small bowel follow-through, enteroclysis, radionuclide studies, angiography, endoscopy.

In the evaluation of these patients, contrastography with barium is of limited diagnostic utility; in particular with *small bowel follow-through*, it is only possible to visualize gross lesions, and the source of bleeding is identified

Table 1. Causes of small bowel bleeding

Vascular lesions	Small bowel tumors	Other causes
Angiodysplasia	Adenoma[2]	Von Willebrand's disease
Dieulafoy's lesion	Hamartoma[3]	Drug-induced small bowel injury
Varices	Lipoma	Diverticulosis
Phlebectasia	Leiomyoma	Meckel's diverticulum
Aortoenteric fistula	Neurofibroma[4]	Crohn's disease
Vasculitis	Neurilemmoma	Amyloidosis
Teleangiectasia[1]	Paraganglioma	Radiation enteritis
	Ganglioneuroma	Zollinger-Ellison syndrome
	Lymphangioma	Infectious causes
	Hemangioma[5]	Ischemic injury
	Islet cell tumor	Ulcers in celiac sprue
	Adenocarcinoma	Chronic ulcerative jejunoileitis
	Lymphoma	Small bowel endometriosis and deciduosis
	Leiomyosarcoma	Pancreaticus hemosuccus/hemobilia
	Angiosarcoma	
	Malignant schwannoma	
	Carcinoid tumor	
	Metastasis	

Associated syndromes: [1]Osler-Weber-Rendu disease, CREST syndrome, Turner's syndrome; [2]FAP; [3]Peutz-Jeghers syndrome; [4]Von Recklinghausen's disease; [5]Blue rubber bleb nevus syndrome, Klippel-Trenaunay-Weber syndrome in only 5% of investigations. With enteroclysis, the percentage may reach 20%.

Scintigraphy and selective angiography of the mesenteric district are used in cases of massive blood loss.

Scintigraphy with red cells marked with Tc99 is used when bleeding is distal to the duodenojejunal angle of Treiz. Unfortunately, although it is possible to identify the small bowel as the seat of bleeding, it is not possible to diagnose the exact location. Furthermore, delayed investigation, performed 12-24 h after injecting the marker, can be deceptive, since it identifies the area of blood flow aspecifically. In the opinion of some researchers, the method is of no use either as an investigation preliminary to angiography or as a surgical guide.

Scintigraphy with Tc99 pertechnetate is useful in patients with OGIB to diagnose Meckel's diverticulum; the sensitivity of the test is 75-100%.

Selective angiography of the mesenteric district can reveal bleeding when it is of 0.5 ml/min. With this technique, bleeding can be diagnosed in 50%-86% of patients with massive bleeding, but the percentage drops to 25%-50% if bleeding is slower or has ceased. If an angiographically suspect area is detected, it may be useful to inject methylene blue during surgical exploration, so that the surgeon can better identify the segment involved and limit surgical resection. Injection of vasoconstrictors, or embolization of the terminal vessels, sometimes makes it possible to control bleeding.

In evaluating the source of obscure bleeding, it is mandatory that the small bowel be endoscopically investigated.

In the literature, *push enteroscopy* reveals the site or probable cause of bleeding in from 40% to 80% of cases. Therapeutic interventions, such as coagulation of vascular malformations or polypectomy, can be accomplished during the procedure (Table 2).

Table 2. Push enteroscopy: obscure gastrointestinal bleeding

AUTHOR	PATIENTS	DIAGNOSTIC YIELD (%)	LESIONS WITHIN REACH OF EGD (%)
BARKIN (1992)	28	75	50
HARRIS (1994)	31	61	36
BARKIN (1994)	20	80	63
CHONG (1994)	55	66	60
DAVIES (1995)	11	45	20
CAVE (1995)	69	49	40
VILLAGOMEZ (1996)	42	74	80
PORTWOOD (1996)	41	50	70
SCHMIT (1996)	83	59	20
O' MAHONY (1996)	39	62	18
ZAMAN (1997)	84	40	76
CHAK (1997)	129	70	50
HERRERA (1997)	95	44	33
VAKIL (1997)	29	62	31
PERSONAL EXPERIENCE (1997)	151	48	10

EGD: esophagogastroduodenoscopy

However, it is striking that, in most studies reported, the lesions discovered using push enteroscopy are actually within reach of a skillfully employed standard gastroscope; the extent of the pathology that was missed during previous gastroscopic examinations, perfomed several times in many of these patients, is from 10% to 80% of positive findings at push enteroscopy.

Gastroduodenal vascular malformations, large hiatal hernias with Cameron's lesions, gastroduodenal ulcers, and watermelon stomach are the UGI lesions most frequently missed at esophagogastroduodenoscopy (EGD). The evanescent character of vascular malformations may explain why investigation sometimes remains non-diagnostic; nevertheless, proper clinical interpretation of abnormalities seen in patients with OGIB is of primary importance.

Since push enteroscopy is an intensive and costly procedure, patients should be more carefully selected for submission to enteroscopy. It would therefore be prudent to repeat EGD before referring the patient for enteroscopy. In general, such "proximal lesions" should be prop-

Table 3. Sonde enteroscopy: obscure gastrointestinal bleeding

AUTHOR	PATIENTS	DIAGNOSTIC YIELD (%)
LEWIS (1988)	60	33
BARTHEL (1990)	18	28
RADEMAKER (1991)	23	30
GOSTOUT (1991)	35	26
VAN GOSSUM (1992)	17	28
MORRIS (1992)	65	38
SCHLAUCH (1993)	27	22
GOLDSTEIN (1994)	27	41
BERNER (1994)	553	58*
CONN (1995)	29	61*
BENZ (1996)	52	15

* Results mixed with push

erly evaluated during EGD and treated if they are clinically relevant. If symptoms do not resolve after treatment, the patient should undergo push enteroscopy.

With *sonde enteroscopy* in patients with OGIB, the diagnostic yield varies from 15% to 41%; however, no therapeutic intervention is possible. In a large retrospective case study of patients with OGIB, both push and sonde enteroscopy was evaluated, and a diagnostic success rate of 58% was reported (Table 3).

Also, with the use of sonde enteroscopy, angiodysplasias were the most frequent finding (80%), while neoplasias did not exceed 10%. This method has also been used to evaluate patients with OGIB undergoing treatment with NSAID, in whom a high incidence of ulceration of the small bowel has been detected.

Lastly, with intraoperative enteroscopy, identification of the source of bleeding is possible in 70%-100% of cases. During this procedure it is possible to coagulate isolated vascular malformations, whereas surgical resection is indicated in the case of neoplasias or sporadic vascular lesions that do not involve the small bowel diffusely. Moreover, long-term follow-up of patients with OGIB in whom intraoperative enteroscopy has been performed has shown that about 30% experience a further episode of bleeding.

Diagnostic approach in patients with OGIB

The patient with chronic unexplained bleeding can be a source of frustration, from the standpoints of establishing diagnosis and managing blood loss, especially if the bleeding continues to remain obscure after exhaustive tests.

The clinical history in a patient with OGIB may suggest a possible cause, but is rarely diagnostic; however, a bleeding dyscrasia should always be considered in patients with recurrent bleeding. The extent of evaluation required for the patient with OGIB depends on the severity of bleeding and the patient's age (Fig. 1).

If massive blood loss continues after suitable intensive care, a gastroduodenal or colonic cause must be ruled out by performing EGD immediately, followed by total colonoscopy with exploration of the terminal ileum. It is equally important to achieve correct visualization of the papilla of Vater, using a side-viewing duodenoscope, to exclude bleeding from the bileopancreatic tract. Selective mesenteric arteriography must be used in cases unresolved by the preceding investigations. During an arrest of bleeding, even if temporary, push enteroscopy may be diagnostic (Fig. 2 a-c).

Surgery with intraoperative enteroscopy is necessary when bleeding persists and is transfusion-dependent. Methods such as scintigraphy or intraoperative arteriography are useful to locate the source of bleeding precisely and limit resection of the small bowel.

If a patient has both persistent transfusion-dependent bleeding and a high surgical risk, sonde enteroscopy may be a worthwhile investigation to aid in the decision as to whether surgery must be performed. This procedure should only be carried out by an experienced endoscopist and team in an istitution where the procedure is routinely done. In the future, more

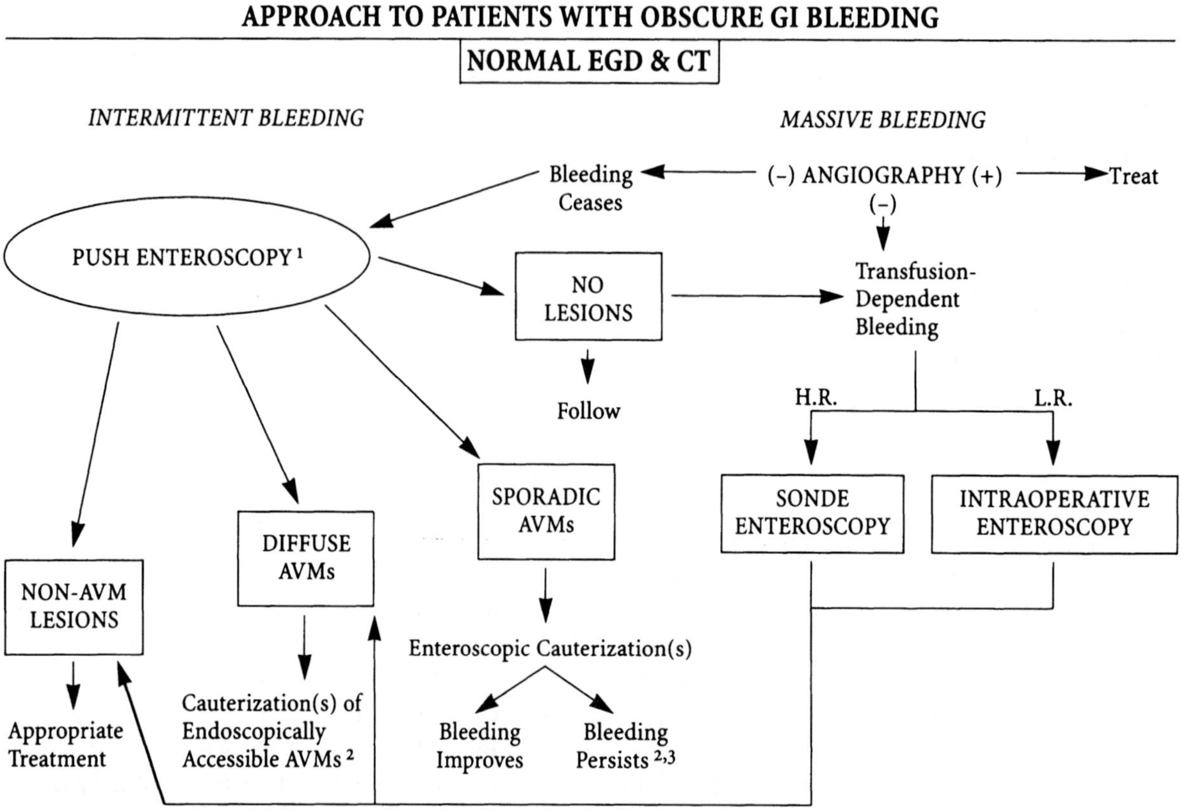

APPROACH TO PATIENTS WITH OBSCURE GI BLEEDING

NORMAL EGD & CT

Fig. 1. (1) Enteroclysis: Meckel's scan on laparoscopy is advocated in patients under 50 years in whom small bowel tumors and Meckel's diverticulum are most likely; (2) add medical treatment: octreotide, estrogen-progesterone, iron replacement therapy; (3) perform intraoperative enteroscopy in selected patients

EGD: esophagogastroduodenoscopy; CT: total colonoscopy; AVMs: vascular malformations; H.R.: high risk for surgery; L.R.: low risk for surgery

innovative applications of enteroscopy, such as laparoscopically assisted total enteroscopy, may allow complete examination of the small bowel to be associated with an immediate means of minimally invasive extirpative therapy, thus avoiding the undesirable aspects of open laparatomy.

When bleeding is intermittent, however, and where the only clinical datum is heme-positive stool with anemia, in consideration of its high diagnostic efficiency and therapeutic possibilities, push enteroscopy should be performed early, as the first investigation after EGD and total colonoscopy. Since small bowel angiodysplasias, the most common cause for OGIB, usually tend to be encountered just beyond the distal duodenum and the proximal jejunum, it should be stressed that the distal duodenum and the first jejunal loop may also be adequately investigated with a less cumbersome and less costly procedure, for example with a 118-cm-long esophagogastroduodenoscope (personal observation). Moreover, in young patients, below the age of 50, in whom tumor of the small bowel is the most frequent cause of OGIB, push enteroscopy should be associated with enteroclysis to exclude gross sources of bleeding in areas of the small bowel that cannot be reached endoscopically. Alternatively, double-way enteroscopy may be used. In young patients, Meckel's diverticulum should also be excluded via a Meckel's scan. A CT scan of the abdomen and pelvis should be done to complete the screening for macroscopic vascular or neoplastic abnormalities. Benign neoplasms or Meckel's diverticulum may also be identified and resected laparoscopically in selected patients.

However, despite the use of all the available diagnostic methods, in about 30%-40% of patients the cause of bleeding is not identified. In addition, the ultimate impact of diagnostic and/or therapeutic enteroscopy on the actual

Atlas of Enteroscopy

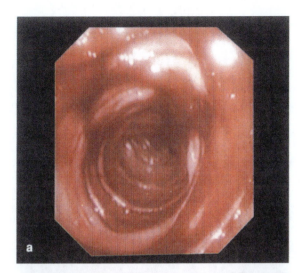

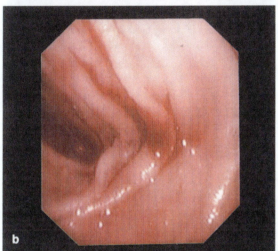

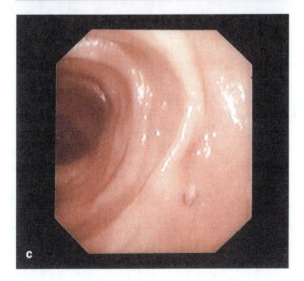

Fig. 2. a Massive small bowel bleeding. b The suspect bleeding source has been identified in the first jeunal loop. c Result after heater probe cauterization of a Dieulafoy's lesion

clinical outcome for the patient with OGIB remains to be determined. In spite of the ability to find a probable cause of bleeding in the small bowel by various techniques and to apply appropriate treatment, the rate of recurrent bleeding remains significant.

Suggested reading

Pennazio M, Rossini FP (1998) Main issues in push enteroscopy. Ital J Gastroenterol Hepatol 30:96-101

Peterson WL (1988) Obscure gastrointestinal bleeding. Med Clin N Am 72:1169-1176

Rossini FP, Arrigoni A, Pennazio M (1996) Clinical enteroscopy. J Clin Gastroenterol 22:231-236

Angiodysplasias

A. Van Gossum, A. Schmit

Gastrointestinal bleeding is a common problem and represents a major cause of morbidity and mortality. Annual rates of approximately 125 episodes per 100,000 inhabitants are suggested by population-based studies from the 1960s and 1970s. In about 5% of patients with digestive blood loss, no bleeding site is identified after routine upper and lower endoscopy and small bowel X-ray series. In these cases, a small bowel origin of the bleeding has to be suspected. Many causes of intestinal bleeding have to be considered. However, before considering a small bowel origin, upper or lower gastrointestinal bleeding has to be excluded with certainty.

Several terms like arteriovenous malformations, vascular ectasias, vascular malformations or angiomas are currently used to describe angiodysplasias (AD). Standardization of endoscopic or pathologic description of AD within the gut is still missing.

Two major types of AD have to be distinguished: (a) hereditary AD in Weber-Osler-Rendu disease and (b) acquired AD. Acquired AD appear typically in older patients. These submucosal collections of dilated capillaries and veins develop secondary to prolonged intermittent obstruction of venous outflow. The chronic obstruction leads to increased backpressure in the capillary bed, resulting in incompetence of the prearteriolar sphincters and development of small arteriovenous shunts. The mucosa overlying these small shunts may receive an inadequate blood supply, resulting in localized ischemia with ulceration and subsequent bleeding.

Although an association between AD and several diseases such as aortic stenosis, renal insufficiency or Von Willebrand's disease has been described, no direct relationship has been proven.

Vascular malformations have been recognized as an important cause of both chronic and acute blood loss. The clinical manifestations of patients with gastrointestinal AD are variable, ranging from occult blood loss to melena. The feature of blood loss is not likely to help the clinician in making a differential diagnosis. Patients often suffer from microcytic anemia and blood transfusion needs may be considerable.

Investigation procedures

AD do not distort the mucosa, and so they are missed by barium studies. Thus, AD have to be differentiated from hemangiomas, which are tumorlike lesions. Angiography-based diagnosis of AD is not fully reliable because the AD may be too small to be detected by angiography. This examination should be performed when the lesion is bleeding actively, with a bleeding rate of at least 0.5 ml/min. Furthermore, the small bowel usually requires superselective catheterization to localize hemorrhage in this location. Isotopic investigations lack specificity, and exact location of the bleeding site is often difficult.

AD are best diagnosed by enteroscopy and they account for 20%-50% of the lesions discovered by this investigation in patients suffering from obscure digestive bleeding. Thus diagnosis of AD is essentially based upon direct visualization by endoscopy. Two major types of enteroscopes are used. The first is a sonde enteroscope, which enables complete intubation of the small bowel, but has no video capacities and has no operating channel. The second type is the video push enteroscope, providing an operating channel, but visualization of the small bowel is limited to the jejunum. Less frequently, the push enteroscope may also be passed through the anus in order to visualize the ileum. Still more exceptional, the enteroscope may be introduced into the gut during a surgical procedure (peroperative enteroscopy). This procedure enables submucosal AD to be visualized by transillumination of the small bowel wall. The overall efficacy of the two types of enteroscopes seems to be comparable. Despite the fact that enteroscopy is considered to be best tool to diagnose AD, some important pitfalls should be highlighted. First, AD may vanish at the moment of the examination. Thus, some investigations remain non-diagnostic despite complete intubation of the small bowel, as may happen with the sonde enteroscope. Second, AD have to be differentiated from traumatic lesions caused by the intubation procedure. Biopsy samples may help to define lesions of uncertain nature, but histology is not always reliable. In addition, it must be pointed out that the risk of performing biopsy of AD is not negligible.

Endoscopic appearence of AD

AD are characterized by three major aspects: (1) the size of the AD; (2) the number of AD; (3) the hemorrhagic feature of AD. The size of AD may vary considerably. Three types of AD can be distinguished: (a) minute AD (less than 2 mm), (b) intermediate AD (from 2 to 5 mm) and (c) large AD (greater than 5 mm). However, it is important to recognize that the apparent part of an AD may only represent the top of an iceberg, because the submucosal part is hidden. Furthermore, as stated before, AD may be completely submerged by the mucosa. Concerning the number of AD, they may either appear as a single lesion, multiple AD (2-10 AD), or they may involve in a diffuse manner the entire small bowel (more than 10 AD). Diffuse AD often imply therapeutic difficulties in coagulating all AD. The fact that some AD spontaneously bleed during enteroscopy or start bleeding after the first attempt at coagulation probably suggests that the lesion was really responsible for the bleeding. Furthermore, AD may present with an pseudoulcerated shape or AD may be surrounded by a fibrinlike deposit. These signs probably indicate recent bleeding events. Furthermore, it may happen that coagulation reveals that the treated AD was much bigger than estimated by the endoscopic appearence.

Treatment

The treatment of AD is still a matter of debate. The natural history may be spontaneously favorable in up to 50% of acquired AD. In Rendu-Osler patients, estroprogestatives have been successfully used, but in patients with acquired AD, estroprogestatives have failed to show clear beneficial effects and are responsible for potentially serious side effects. Push enteroscopy enables cauterization of AD either by argon laser or bicap. Nevertheless, it remains unclear whether or not cauterization changes the natural history of AD. It is also questionable if cauterization AD is really helpful. Controlled studies are mandatory to give a definite answer to the question of how to treat small bowel angiodysplasias.

Suggested reading

Schmit A, Gay F, Adler M, Cremer M, Van Gossum A (1996) Diagnostic efficacy of push-enteroscopy and long term follow-up of patients with small bowel angiodysplasias. Digest Dis Sc 41:2348-2352

Waye J (1997) Enteroscopy. Gastrointest Endosc 46:247-256

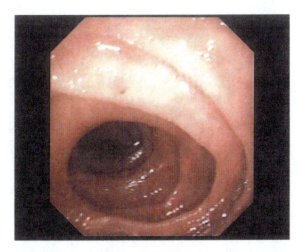

Fig. 1. Minute isolated small bowel AD

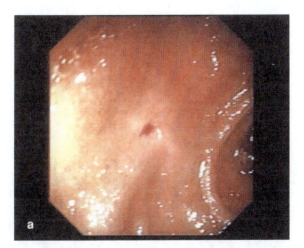 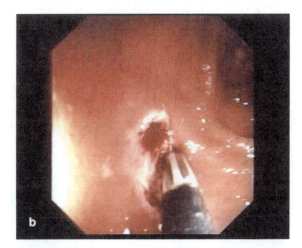

Fig. 2. *Intermediate small bowel AD.* **a** Mildly depressed AD (intermediate size). **b** Transient bleeding of this lesion during coagulation with a bicap probe

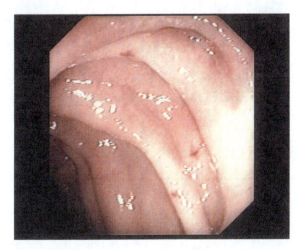

Fig. 3. *Diffuse small bowel AD.* An example of diffuse small bowel AD in a patient with Rendu-Osler disease

Angiodysplasias

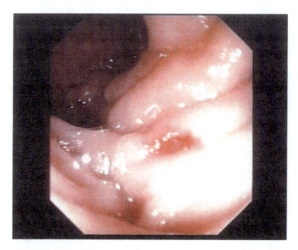

Fig. 4. *Large small bowel AD.* Even a large AD may be hidden between two intestinal folds

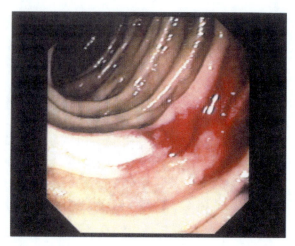

Fig. 5. *Bleeding small bowel AD.* Spontaneous bleeding of an ulcerated AD

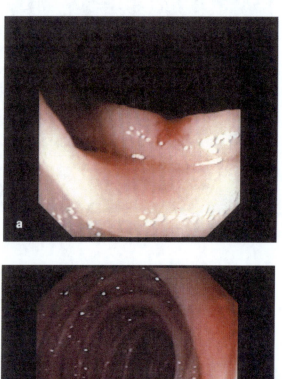

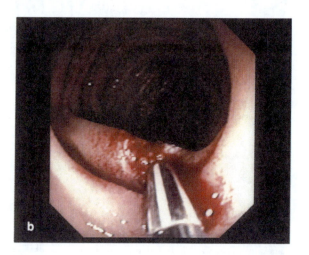

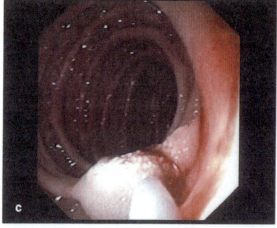

Fig. 6. *Small bowel AD.* a Ulcerated form of a large AD. b Active bleeding during coagulation confirming the bleeding capacity of this lesion. c Submucosal injection of diluted adrenaline through a catheter needle facilitating bleeding control

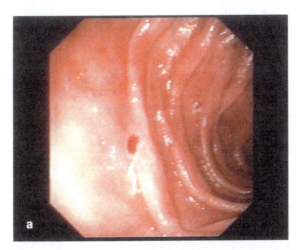 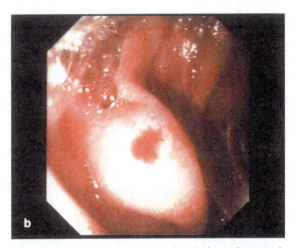

Fig. 7. *Small bowel AD.* **a** Pseudoulcerated shape of a large AD. **b** The size of the AD is better visualized after submucosal injection of diluted adrenaline that has been injected before electrocoagulation

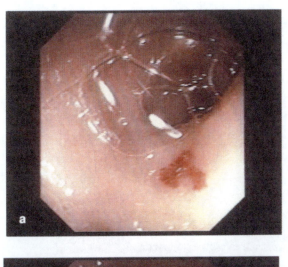

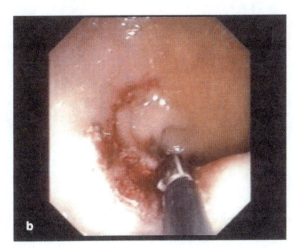

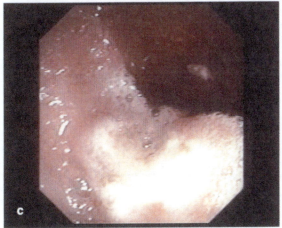

Fig. 8. *Small bowel AD.* **a** Irregular aspect of a large but superficial AD. **b** Per-coagulation bleeding. **c** Endoscopic appearance after coagulation. At this stage, no more vessel is visible

NSAID enteropathy

A.J. Morris

Damage to the gastrointestinal mucosa by non-steroidal anti-inflammatory drugs (NSAID) is the most common iatrogenic disease known to man. The term "NSAID enteropathy" describes a specific small intestinal disease caused by NSAID. It is increasingly recognized that small bowel damage caused by these drugs can result in significant morbidity and mortality in patients with arthritis. Recognition that NSAID gastrointestinal damage extends beyond the distal duodenum has allowed clinicians to improve management of these patients with appropriate investigation and treatment. Small bowel endoscopy has proven pivotal in the investigation of patients with suspected NSAID enteropathy and has allowed studies of early pathological changes of NSAID enteropathy in man.

While the upper gastrointestinal lesions caused by NSAID are well demonstrated, there is increasing evidence of NSAID toxicity to the small bowel. Indirect studies of small bowel damage using 51 chromium EDTA and 111-indium-labelled leukocytes detected inflammation in an estimated 70% of patients on long-term therapy with NSAID. The pathological correlation with these results is currently unknown. A highly selected group of patients with the highest III-indium-labelled leukocyte excretion had small bowel radiology with ulcers detected in 3 of 18 patients examined. In post-mortem studies 8.4% of patients on long-term NSAID had small bowel ulcers, but smaller lesions were probably missed due to inability to preserve specimens in this study. In a review of NSAID enteropathy, it was found that there was a preponderance of females and patients who had been on long-term therapy in case reports of NSAID small bowel damage. There have also been case reports where short-term NSAID ingestion has led to ulceration, emphasizing that dose and formulation may be important in pathogenesis of lesions. Damage from NSAID can persist for many months after withdrawal of the drug, emphasizing the need for retrospective drug history in patients with unexplained small bowel ulceration.

Clinical features

NSAID small bowel ulceration represents a silent epidemic as patients usually have no symptoms until they develop a complication of the disease. A high index of suspicion is needed in a patient who develops unexplained diarrhea, abdominal pain, weight loss or, more commonly, evidence of blood loss. The main complications are iron-deficiency anemia, acute gastrointestinal hemorrhage and small bowel obstruction or perforation.

Iron-deficiency anemia
Using technetium-99-labelled red blood cells, patients receiving NSAID have documented blood loss that is equivalent to that found in

colon cancer. While many clinicians accept the blood loss from gastroduodenal lesions caused by NSAID, the small bowel may be the major site of blood loss in patients on these drugs. In a study from our unit, only 45% of patients on NSAID were found to have an upper GI cause for anemia. Surprisingly, the anemia persisted in 55% of patients after healing of the original lesion, suggesting that over 75% of patients had blood loss from alternative gastrointestinal sites. The suggestion of small bowel bleeding was later confirmed by studies comparing upper gastrointestinal endoscopy findings and fecal blood-loss results.

Acute gastrointestinal hemorrhage

A less common presentation is with melena and hemodynamic upset secondary to acute bleeding. Some patients require emergency laparatomy and segmental resection to control bleeding. In a retrospective study, Langman found that small bowel hemorrhage and perforation were more than twice as frequent in NSAID patients than age-and sex-matched controls.

Small bowel obstruction and perforation

Characteristic small bowel lesions known as "diaphragm" strictures have been reported in patients on long-term NSAID. These abnormalities have been observed in the right hemicolon and can progress to cause critical narrowing and obstruction. Such strictures should be considered in any patient on NSAID with unexplained abdominal pain or signs to suggest obstruction.

Pathophysiology

Early studies of the pathophysiology of NSAID small bowel damage relied on animal models where rats were fed a supraphysiological dose of NSAID. These studies highlighted the fact that NSAID damage was a multifactorial process affected by host factors such as stress, feeding, presence of luminal bacteria and that enterohepatic circulation of the NSAID predisposes to ulceration. Local factors such as topical concentration of NSAID are also important in the disease process. Early pathological events include microvascular occlusion, smooth muscle changes, neutrophil invasion and subsequent ulceration. No long-term administration studies or adjuvant arthritis model studies have been carried out, so these results must be extrapolated to man with great caution.

Human studies

Using intestinal permeability to 51 chromium EDTA and polyethylene glycol 400 as surrogate markers for small bowel integrity, it can be demonstrated that small bowel dysfunction occurs in patients receiving NSAID.

Bjarnason has proposed a two-step process of NSAID damage. Initial mitochondrial damage renders the cells energy-deficient, with subsequent loss of tight junction function. This allows luminal antigen absorption with secondary inflammatory reaction in the mucosa and ulceration in some patients. This hypothesis has still to be fully tested in man.

Pathology of NSAID enteropathy

Prior to the introduction of enteroscopy, little was known about the pathological features of NSAID enteropathy. Case reports confirmed the presence of non-specific ulceration of jejunum and ileum.

A clinicopathological study demonstrated discrete mucosal "diaphragm" strictures characterized by submucosal fibrosis and luminal ulceration in patients on NSAID. A prospective post-mortem study clearly showed ulcers in patients on long-term NSAID, although autolysis of specimens prevented clear assessment of histological changes in patients without ulcers. In a study from our unit using push enteroscopy in patients receiving NSAID, we found both ulceration and subtle microscopic changes.

The NSAID group had inflammatory cell infiltrate, villous blunting and microerosions in areas of macroscopically normal mucosa.

Enteroscopy and NSAID enteropathy

Experience suggests that small bowel radiology is a poor method of detecting NSAID enteropathy. Our initial experience of using sonde enteroscopy in a highly selected population of patients with rheumatoid arthritis and anaemia showed mucosal red spot lesions with ulceration identified in 47% of patients examined. In a larger series the yield remained high, although other authors found less damage using a push enteroscope probably due to the proximal limitation of this technique. Enteroscopy has now identified the earliest mucosal lesions of NSAID enteropathy and will allow further understanding of the pathogenesis of this disease in the future.

NSAID enteropathy is a major cause of morbidity in patients receiving these drugs. Enteroscopy has identified specific small bowel lesions caused by the drugs. Pathophysiological studies using enteroscopy as a method to directly study NSAID toxicity will facilitate development of new treatments for this disease.

Suggested reading

Morris AJ, Potter V, Capell HA, Sturrock RD, Lee FD, MacKenzie JF (1995) Jejunal lesions in human non steroidal anti inflammatory drug (NSAID) enteropathy. Gut 36[Suppl 1]:T153

Morris AJ, Madhok R, Sturrock RD, Capell HA, MacKenzie JF (1991) Enteroscopic diagnosis of small bowel ulceration in patients receiveng non steroidal anti inflamatory drugs. Lancet 337:520

Morris AJ, Wasson LA, MacKenzie JF (1992) Small bowel enteroscopy in undiagnosed gastrointestinal blood loss. Gut 33:887-889

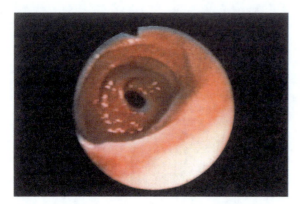

Fig. 1. Enteroscopic view of diaphragm structure

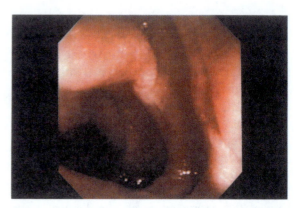

Fig. 2. Typical enteroscopic appearance NSAID enteropathy. Ulceration of jejunal folds

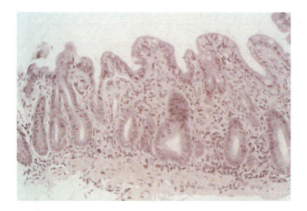

Fig. 3. Villous blunting in jejunum of patient on NSAID

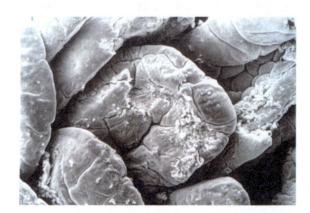

Fig. 4. Electron micrograph of microlesions on jejunal villi

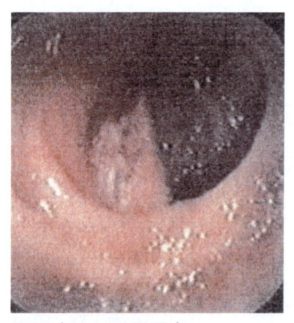

Fig. 5. Push enteroscopy: NSAID ulcer
(by courtesy of Prof. G. Gay, Nancy)

Meckel's diverticulum - Jejunoileal diverticulosis

A. Arrigoni, F.P. Rossini

Jejunoileal diverticula can be divided into two broad categories: *congenital*, present at birth and related to abnormalities of embryologic development, such as Meckel's diverticulum, and *acquired*, which include all others, especially when diffuse and with presentation in adulthood.

Meckel's diverticulum

Meckel's diverticulum is the most frequent congenital abnormality of the intestinal tract, involving 2% of the population, and is the result of an incomplete obliteration of the vitelline duct whose intestinal end persists as a sac.

The diverticulum arises from the antimesenteric border of the ileum, usually within 100 cm of the ileocecal junction, and it varies from 2 to 10 cm in length; the mouth of the sac is large, often being equal to the intestinal lumen itself. Ectopic gastric mucosa lining is frequently encountered in the diverticulum, but pancreatic, colonic and endometrial ectopic tissue has occasionally been described.

Although usually asymptomatic, Meckel's diverticulum may present as lower gastrointestinal bleeding from ulceration of the ileal mucosa adjacent to ectopic gastric mucosa, intestinal obstruction due to intussusception of the diverticulum, volvolus or adhesions or diverticulitis, gangrene and perforation caused by impacted enteroliths, mimicking acute appendicitis.

Approach tests

Radionuclide imaging
If a Meckel's diverticulum is suspected, abdominal scanning after administration of Tc-99m, which is concentrated by parietal cell-containing ectopic gastric mucosa, is the study of choice.

Radiology
Only infrequently can a diagnosis of Meckel's diverticulum be made by X-ray study. Gas filling the diverticulum or a large opaque enterolith may occasionally be recognized on plain film of the abdomen. Barium may fill the diverticulum at enteroclysis.

Endoscopy
As Meckel's diverticulum is distally located in the ileum, it is an unusual endoscopic finding, both at push or sonde enteroscopy and at retrograde ileoscopy. Intraoperative enteroscopy, performed in patients with gastrointestinal bleeding of obscure origin, can occasionally identify a previously undetected Meckel's diverticulum as the source of bleeding.

Definitive diagnosis
The diagnostic test is abdominal scanning after administration of Tc-99m, although false-negative and false-positive results have been reported.

Jejunoileal diverticulosis

Is a heterogeneous disorder characterized by the presence of multiple diverticula that are mostly jejunal but can be also present in the duodenum and ileum? Though the pathogenesis remains poorly understood, small bowel diverticula are caused by disorders of the smooth muscle and myenteric plexus. Whether they represent separate disorders or whether they are manifestations of either progressive systemic sclerosis or visceral myopathy is unknown. Radiological studies report a prevalence of 0.5%-5% and the incidence increases with age.

Jejunal diverticula are lined with mucosa, muscolaris mucosae and submucosa. In myopathies fibrosis of the muscular layer causes localized areas of atrophy and weakness, which then protrude, creating sacculation. In contrast, in disorders of the myenteric plexus, it is possible that uncoordinated motility creates areas of increased intraluminal pressure, with protrusion of the mucosa and submucosa along defects at the point of blood-vessel penetration.

Only 10%-40% of patients with jejunoileal diverticulosis are symptomatic. When symptoms are present they are often those of chronic intestinal pseudo-obstruction. The diverticula may become complicated by acute inflammation, perforation or bleeding. True mechanical obstruction secondary to inflammation, adhesions, enteroliths and volvulus can also complicate jejunoileal diverticulosis. The underlying ineffective motility may result in a stagnant loop syndrome, with diarrhea, steatorrhea or megaloblastic anemia. In these patients bacterial overgrowth can be demonstrated by the culture of properly collected aspirates from the proximal intestine.

Approach tests

Radiology
Air-fluid levels are seen at upright plain abdomen in patients with jejunoileal diverticulosis. Barium contrast series can demonstrate larger diverticula, but the smaller ones can escape detection because of scarce filling or distortion due to extrinsic compression. Therefore, a negative examination does not exclude jejunoileal diverticulosis. Enteroclysis is thought to be more sensitive and can improve the diagnosis. CT scan can be useful in selected cases.

Endoscopy
Push enteroscopy or sonde enteroscopy may occasionally reveal jejunal diverticula. Besides the direct observation of diverticula, in patients with suspected bacterial overgrowth, push enteroscopy permits a quick collection of juice specimens at different levels along the jejunum. On the other hand, forcep biopsies taken during enteroscopy are of no aid for the diagnosis of neuropathy or myopathy, as these require full-thickness surgical biopsies.

Definitive diagnosis
Enteroclysis is the most reliable diagnostic method for the diagnosis of jejunoileal diverticulosis. Jejunoileal diverticula are often an occasional finding during laparotomy performed for different reasons.

Suggested reading

Cooney DR, Duszenski DO, Camboa E, Karp MP, Jeweit DC (1982) The abdominal technectium scan (a decade of experience). J Pediatr Surg 17:611-619

Maglinte D, Chernish S, DeWeese R (1986) Acquired jejunoileal diverticular disease: subject review. Radiology 158:577-580

Soltero MJ, Bill AH (1976) The natural history of Meckel's diverticulum and its relations to incidental removal. Am J Surgery 132:168-173

Atlas of Enteroscopy

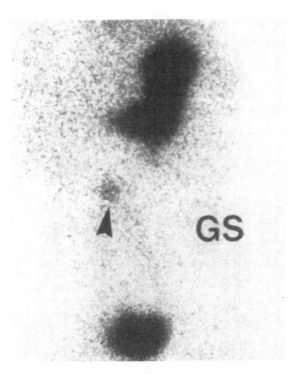

Fig. 1. *Meckel's diverticulum.* Technectium-99m scan of Meckel's diverticulum demonstrating ectopic uptake in an area (*arrowhead*) superior to the bladder and inferior to the stomach in the anterior projection

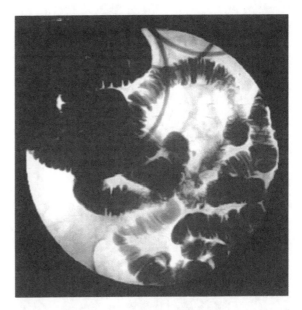

Fig. 2. *Meckel's diverticulum.* Enteroclysis: ulcerated Meckel's diverticulum with accessory sack (by courtesy of Dr. E. Juliani, Turin, Italy)

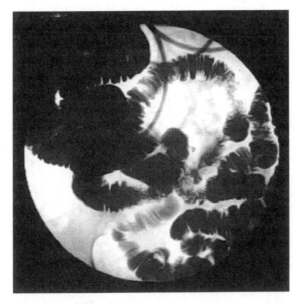

Fig. 3. *Jejunoileal diverticulosis.* Enteroclysis: multiple sacklike barium-filled defects protruding from the intestinal lumen, consistent with jejuno-ileal diverticulosis (by courtesy of Dr. E. Juliani, Turin, Italy)

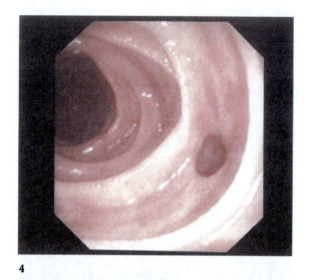
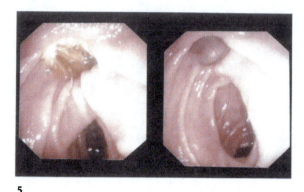
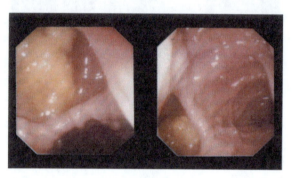

Figs. 4-6. *Jejunoileal diverticulosis.* Endoscopic appearance of jejunal diverticula seen during push enteroscopy

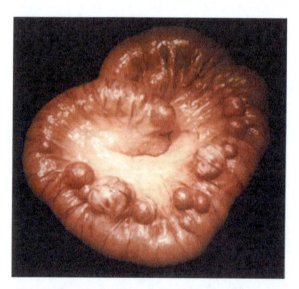

Fig. 7. *Jejunoileal diverticulosis.* Multiple outpouchings along the mesenteric border of jejunum characteristic of jejunal diverticulosis, occasionally observed at laparotomy

DIARRHEA AND MALABSORPTION

Diarrhea and malabsorption syndromes: clinic overview

Diarrhea and malabsorption: the role of enteroscopy

Coeliac disease

Tropical sprue

Whipple's disease

Ulcerative jejunoileitis

Eosinophilic enteropathy

Vasculitis

Crohn's disease

Amyloidosis

Sarcoidosis

Mastocytosis

Abeta and hypobetalipoproteinemias

Hypogammaglobulinemia

Diarrhea and malabsorption syndromes: clinical overview

P. Mainguet

The indications of enteroscopy in malabsorption syndromes are relatively limited with regard to investigations in cases of occult bleeding in the digestive tract and in detecting benign or malignant lesions of the small intestine. Nevertheless, extensive proximal push enteroscopy with detailed examination of a large area of the jejunum contributes to the differential diagnosis of chronic diarrhea or malabsorption syndrome both in children or adults. A unit of gastroenterology adequately equipped for push enteroscopy can be considered effective if it fulfills the following items:

- A high score of correct enteroscopic diagnoses corresponding to an appropriate selection of patients
- Optimal use of the possibilities offered by enteroscopy, i.e., samples for a complementary immunohistochemical examination, fluid for bacterial counts
- Good patient compliance with regard to further enteroscopies
- A worthwhile cost/benefit ratio as a result of fulfilling the above conditions and avoiding multiple, expensive biological tests and functional examinations that are less sensitive or less specific than the endoscopic examination itself. As yet, the cost/benefit ratio is unknown, because of the relative rarity of indications and the lack of multicentric studies.

When confronted with chronic diarrhea, the first step towards a diagnosis is to look at the clinical data and conduct simple, cheap examinations. The frequency of bowel movements is an imprecise criterion and can be confused with repeated afecal stools or anorectal continence disorders. On the other hand, the timetable of passing stools, their relationship to meals, or the possible decrease in diarrhea during a period of fasting are all relevant signs:

- Nocturnal diarrhea causing the patient to awaken always has an organic origin
- Postprandial diarrhea preceded by meteorism, abdominal colic relieved by breaking wind, points to an osmotic diarrhea which stops during temporary withdrawal of food
- Morning diarrhea with successive liquid stools evokes cholegenic diarrhea due to malabsorption of biliary salts, as happens in a lesion of the distal ileum or after its surgical resection
- Uncontrollable diarrhea without any specific timetable, with stools lacking any tissue elements (phlegm, blood, pus) points to secretory (endocrinal causes, laxatives) or motor diarrhea (hyperthyroid)
- Chronic diarrhea (lasting more than 4 weeks) suggests primary malabsorption when it leads to significant loss of weight in a patient free of any known tumor or metabolic disorder who continues to consume sufficient and adequate food.

Two easily performed methods can provide discriminatory parameters contributing to the diagnosis:

- Twenty-four hour fecal output is less than 200 g/24 h if the food intake is unchanged with regard to the period preceding the test
- Measurement of fecal osmolality in the 24 h stool shows an "ion gap."

When osmotic diarrhea is suspected in a patient who does not consume antiacids, the common causes are:
- Consumption of fruit or dietary products
- Sorbitol (20 g/day)
- Lactose intolerance due to primary deficiency

In chronic diarrhea with a fecal output greater than 200 g/24 h, prior to any intestinal morphological examination, the assessment includes: coproculture, stool examination for parasites and research of steatorrhea. The presence of lipids in the stools permits a differential diagnosis between a lipid hydrolysis defect (lipase deficit and/or biliary salts) and an absorption disorder by the intestinal mucosa. When steatorrhea has an intestinal origin, the mean values of water and Na⁺/24 h output are higher than in pancreatic insufficiency. If there is agreement between the clinical data and the above values, the hypothesis of a pancreatic pathology leads, first and foremost, to morphological investigations (CT scan, echoendoscopy, MR imaging, possibly ERCP). Quantitative assessment of a steatorrhea of pancreatic origin can be provided with sufficient sensitivity and specificity by the C_{13} trioleine breathtest.

The diagnostic approach to intestinal pathology is focused on the evidence of morphological abnormalities. In the absence of any detectable steatorrhea, colonoscopy or coloileoscopy is the first approach. In 50% of cases of chronic diarrhea, these methods reveal macroscopic features (inflammatory disorders, ischemic lesions...) or microscopic lesions detected in staged biopsies (collagen colitis, lymphocytic colitis). When a small intestine disease is suspected, the choice of a technique for evaluating the small intestine depends on biological and clinical parameters that will point to either a diffuse disorder of the mucosa or a segmentary disorder.

Diagnosis of malabsorption in absence of chronic diarrhea

Besides the digestive tract, the signs most often observed in celiac disease are: anemia, usually with iron deficiency, complaints due to osteoporosis or osteomalacia. In the blind loop syndrome, a macrocystic anemia can also be the first or the only clinical sign of malabsorption when steatorrhea is absent.

Diagnosis of celiac disease (CD) in routine endoscopy

An iron deficiency, especially in an elderly patient, brings first to mind occult bleeding. Gastroduodenoscopy, carried out in order to find a lesion responsible for sideropenia, enables the careful observer to recognize the mucosal abnormalies suggestive of an untreated CD, reduction in number or absence of Kerckring's folds, mosaic pattern, scalloped folds, or visibility of superficial blood vessels. The association of two or three signs has a sensitivity of 92% to 100% and a specificity of 92% to 97%. Biopsies correctly sampled and in a sufficient number on the face or on the crest folds (when they are present) permit a diagnosis of total villous atrophy (TVA). Nevertheless, in some cases the interpretation of biopsy material from the duodenum remains doubtful. In these patients enteroscopy is useful and should be performed. In practice, the biopsy samples that the majority of pathologists accept as equivalent to biopsies by suction aspiration must satisfy the correctly codified sampling conditions:

- Three biopsies taken on the face or on the crest of the valvulae conniventes permit a conventional histological examination to be made with villometric measurements and IEL counts.
- Two supplementary biopsies permit disaccharidase activities to be measured. These last samples are optional, but a great fall in lactase and sucrase values is a sign usually observed in chronic celiac disease, and the response to treatment is more often than not accompanied by a return to normal or subnormal values of disaccharidase activity.

Serological diagnosis of celiac disease in selected patients

Serological tests have become a cheap, sensitive and selective screening method with a high positive predictive value in the diagnosis of gluten-enteropathy. They cover nearly all untreated adult patients, and recent studies confirm the convergence of resuls, that is to say, a specificity and sensitivity approaching 100% when the IgA anti-endomysium antibodies and the IgA and IgG antigliadine antibodies are positive in a symptomatic adult.

Diagnosis of the blind-loop syndrome

The glucose breath test is an adequate first approach with a sensitivity of 62% and a specificity of 83%. When stasis involves a jejunal loop accessible to enteroscopy (jejunal diverticulosis, gastrectomy with an afferent blind loop, parietal amyloid infiltration), a method of sterile catheterization has been proposed, allowing samples to be obtained for identification and counting of bacteria, as well as assessment of the primary/secondary bile acids ratio. The "gold standard" remains a sample of intestinal liquid and permits the determination of a proliferation of microorganism responsible for biliary salt deconjugation: Eubacteria, Bacteroids, Corynebacteria.

Conclusions

Push enteroscopy provides an important contribution to the diagnosis of chronic diarrhea in the context of malabsorption syndromes. The diagnostic efficiency depends on a stage-to-stage approach based on the clinical data and simple examinations which, if correctly interpreted, will successively eliminate the disorders that do not concern enteroscopy. This approach probably improves the cost/benefit ratio, although this remains to be proved.

Suggested reading

Cerf M (1992) Strategie diagnostique devant une diarrhée chronique de l'adulte. Gastroenterol Clin Biol 16: T12-T21

Diarrhea and malabsorption: the role of enteroscopy

M. Pennazio, F.P. Rossini

Mucosal biopsy is considered the gold standard for the diagnosis of many diseases affecting the small bowel, especially those associated with malabsorption. Diseases such as celiac sprue, Whipple's disease, and abetalipoproteinemia, which affect the small bowel diffusely, are readily diagnosed by biopsy of the small bowel. In taking jejunal biopsies, a suction capsule has been widely used; however, endoscopic duodenal biopsies are now most commonly used in investigating small-bowel histology. Endoscopic specimens are well recognized as being equally adequate as suction-capsule biopsies in the diagnosis of villous atrophy. Nevertheless, intepretation of proximal duodenal biopsy specimens in small bowel disease may be hampered by the normal occurrence of flattened villi and Brunner's glands and by duodenitis, often present but usually irrelevant to any malabsorption process. Multiple biopsies can, of course, be obtained using endoscopic forceps, but since they can only safely be taken from the zone of the distal duodenum within endoscopic view, their value may be limited.

Moreover, diseases such as intestinal lymphoma, lymphangiectasia, dermatitis herpetiformis, eosinophilic enteritis, Crohn's disease and some opportunistic infections may be patchy in their distribution, and biopsy of the proximal small bowel is helpful only if an involved area is sampled.

In the endoscopic diagnostic approach to malabsorption, push enteroscopy, which offers the possibility of inspecting both the duodenum and the jejunum, as well as of obtaining adequate biopsy material in different and more remote areas, has recently been proposed. The high-resolution image provided by modern video enteroscopes makes possible an accurate study of the mucosal pattern. Moreover, vision of minute mucosal details is further enhanced by instilling water to cover the space between the area to be viewed and the tip of the enteroscope; indigo carmine or methylene blue staining emphasizes the pathological mucous pattern, thus enhancing clarity and diagnostic yield; jejunal fluid may also be collected for microbiological analysis (Fig. 1).

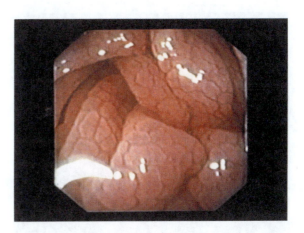

Fig. 1. Endoscopic appearance of normal small bowel mucosa: instillation of water to cover the space between the area to be viewed and the tip of the enteroscope makes possible vision of minute mucosal details (by courtesy of Prof. J. Bures, Hradec Kralowe, Czech Republic)

Few studies have been published concerning the use of enteroscopy in evaluating patients with diarrhea or malabsorption. In the main, patients with suspected celiac disease have been investigated and a diagnosis made only by biopsying the jejunum. Most researchers have concluded that if random proximal mucosal biopsies had been taken, they would probably have revealed the same microscopic changes consistent with celiac sprue. It must be stressed, however, that none of these studies actually made a direct comparison between duodenal and jejunal histology.

In a prospective study, we evaluated whether push enteroscopy improves the diagnostic yield in comparison to an endoscopic exploration restricted to the descending duodenum. Fifty-two patients with diarrhea undiagnosed by routine investigation, or in whom malabsorption was suspected, underwent push enteroscopy. In all patients, at least four biopsies were taken in the descending duodenum and at least four in the jejunum: biopsies were obtained both from mucosa with a normal appearance and from abnormal areas.

Taking the jejunal biopsy as diagnostic standard, the sensitivity of the duodenal biopsy fell to 72%, with a specificity at 100%.

In some cases, the endoscopic mucosal appearance was indicative of small-bowel pathology:

- "Mosaic" mucous pattern consisting of scattered Kerckring's folds that were decreased in height with polygonal areas separated by flat grooves, indicative of subtotal villous atrophy; other endoscopic aspects of the atrophic mucosa, less frequent in our experience, were disappearance of folds and presence of scalloped folds.
- "Glacè icing-like" mucous pattern consisting of increased height of Kerckring's folds with whitish protrusions exuding a milky substance, indicative of lymphangiectasia (Figs. 2-5).

Multiple reports have documented that the abnormalities seen in the duodenum during esophagogastroduodenoscopy (EGD) are sensitive and specific for the detection of patients with malabsorptive disorders such as celiac sprue (see chapter "Celiac disease"). Our data are in agreement with these observations, though absence of these endoscopic duodenal markers of villous atrophy does not exclude that condition. Since in our patients with celiac disease the endoscopic appearance of the mucosa was abnormal both in the duodenum and in the jejunum, it would seem that in cases previously diagnosed by routine EGD, the clinical usefulness of push enteroscopy is doubtful.

Nevertheless, push enteroscopy adds useful information in patients in whom endoscopic/

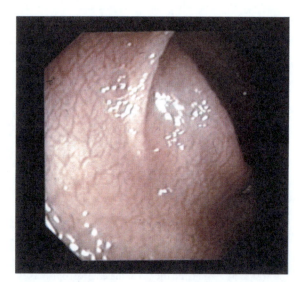

Fig. 2. *Celiac disease*: "mosaic" mucous pattern

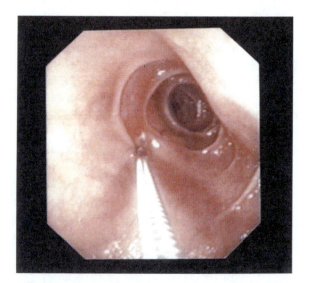

Fig. 3. *Celiac disease*: disappearance of Kerckring's folds at maximal insufflation

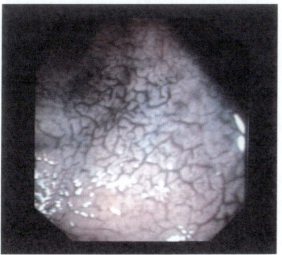

Fig. 4. *Celiac disease*: indigo carmine staining emphasizes the mosaic mucous pattern

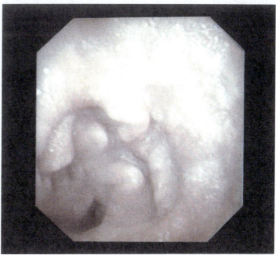

Fig. 5. *Lymphangiectasia*: "glacè icing-like" mucous pattern

histological duodenal findings are inconclusive; it may also be employed to verify correlations between the severity of the clinical picture in celiac disease and the extent of intestinal lesions. Moreover, this technique may be useful to diagnose complications such as ulcerative jejunoileitis or small bowel neoplasia (Tables 1, 2).

Table 1. Endoscopic approach to malabsorption and current indications to enteroscopy

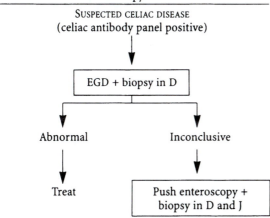

Moreover, analogous to other diseases with patchy involvement, it has been reported that loss of normal villous architecture in celiac disease may be confined to either the proximal or the distal small bowel. Considering the patchy nature of mucosal changes, the diagnosis can be

Table 2. Endoscopic approach to malabsorption and current indications to enteroscopy

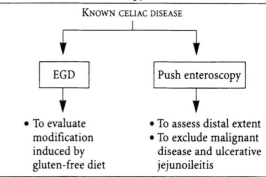

missed if only duodenal or only jejunal biopsies are taken; therefore, a combination of both biopsies, which is feasible with enteroscopy, might increase the diagnostic yield.

In a similar vein, an American study investigated the role of push enteroscopy in evaluating diarrhea in a group of 48 patients with AIDS. In all 9 patients in whom a small bowel source of diarrhea was identified, enteroscopy and jejunal biopsy were both required to make the diagnosis; distal duodenal biopsy alone was not diagnostic in any patient.

In our study we have also observed eight patients, with normal mucosal appearance both in the duodenum and in the jejunum, in whom the diagnosis could on!y be made by biopsying the jejunum. In selected cases, therefore, it could be useful to take multiple biopsies even from mucosa of apparently normal aspect, particularly if there is the clinical suspicion of small bowel mucosal disease.

With the advent of push enteroscopy, further endoscopic exploration and tissue diagnosis of a radiographically suspected disease has become possible. As far as Crohn's disease is concerned, push enteroscopy can correctly evaluate patients with doubtful radiological findings at enteroclysis. When lesions are identified by both techniques, the information obtained is additive: enteroclysis is more effective for distal disease, and in assessing both the extent of the disease and possible complications (fistulas); but enteroscopy allows biopsy for differential diagnosis between Crohn's and other diseases (Iymphoma, ulcerative jejunoileitis, IPSID), and to assess disease activity (Table 3).

Table 3. Endoscopic approach to malabsorption and current indications to enteroscopy

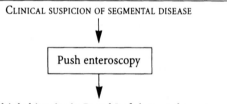

In conclusion, push enteroscopy may be useful in the further diagnosis of difficult cases of diarrhea and malabsorption, since signs indicative of malabsorption can be inspected endoscopically. When abnormal areas or even slight mucosal abnormalities are present, the endoscopist can direct the biopsy forceps to those areas that could be more productive of diagnostic tissue.

With regard to diseases that usually affect the small bowel diffusely, such as celiac disease, EGD with duodenal biopsies is sufficient to make a diagnosis in most patients already suspected of having the disease and push enteroscopy, which is a more expensive procedure, should be reserved for selected patients. Conversely, there is no doubt that when a segmental disease is suspected such as a lymphoma, Crohn's disease, ischemic jejunitis, jejunal vasculitis, eosinophilic enteritis, Iymphangiectasia, or parasitic infections, push enteroscopy could be proposed as first-choice endoscopic examination (Table 3).

Suggested reading

Barkin JS, Schonfeld W, Thomsen S, Manten HD, Rogers AI (1985) Enteroscopy and small bowel biopsy - an improved technique for the diagnosis of small bowel disease. Gastrontest Endosc 31:215-217

Maurino E, Capizzano H, Niveloni S, Kogan Z, Valero J, Boerr L, Bai JC (1993) Value of endoscopic markers in celiac disease. Dig Dis Sci 38 2028-2033

Pennazio M, Arrigoni A, Rossini FP (1996) Push enteroscopy for evaluating patients with diarrhoea or malabsorption. Acta Endosc 26:249-254

Celiac disease

G.R. Corazza, M. Di Stefano, M.A. Pistoia

Celiac disease (non-tropical sprue, gluten-sensitive enteropathy) is a chronic condition in which there is a characteristic, though non-specific, mucosal lesion of the small intestine, which impairs nutrient absorption by the involved bowel, and which improves on withdrawal of wheat gliadins and barley and rye prolamins from the diet.

The clinical presentation of celiac disease is extremely varied, ranging from "classical forms" characterized by the occurrence of diarrhea, steatorrhea, weight loss, abdominal distention, lassitude, and malaise to "subclinical forms" characterized by the presence of minor, transient and extraintestinal symptoms such as anemia, bone pain, spontaneous abortion, infertility, alopecia, or even to "silent forms", more frequently diagnosed among first-degree relatives of celiac patients. Moreover, diagnosis is often suggested by the presence of other conditions known to be associated with celiac disease, such as type I diabetes, thyroid disease, IgA nephropathy, rheumatoid arthritis, Down's syndrome, IgA deficiency, epilepsy with cerebral calcifications.

Approach tests

Radiology
Radiology has practically no role in the diagnosis of uncomplicated, untreated celiac disease, unless intestinal malignancy, strictures or ulcerations are suspected. However, the reduction in number of the jejunal folds together with the increased number of ileal folds, evident at small bowel enema, are considered specific features of this disease (Fig. 1).

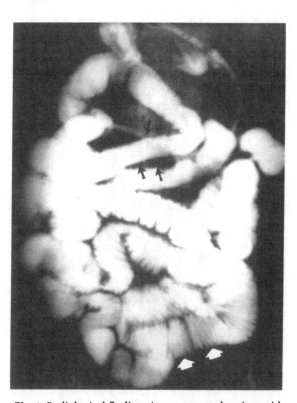

Fig. 1. Radiological findings in an untreated patient with adult celiac disease. Small bowel enema shows reduction in the number of jejunal folds (*black arrows*) together with the increased number of ileal folds (*white arrows*)

Table 1. Sensitivity and specificity of endoscopic markers in celiac disease

	Sensitivity (%)	Specificity (%)
Reduction or loss of Kerckring folds		
Brocchi at al, N Engl Med (1988)	88	83
Mc Intyre et al, Gastrointest Endosc (1992)	73	97
Van Bergeijk et al, J Clin Nutr Gastroenterol (1993)	75	100
Mauriño et al, Dig Dis Sci (1993)	76	98
Scalloped folds		
Jabbari et al, Gastroenterology (1988); adult celiac disease	78	
Corazza et al, Gastrointest Endosc (1993); childhood celiac disease	88	87
Reduction or loss of Kerckring folds + mosaic pattern		
Rossini et al, J Clin Gastroenterol (1996)	92	97
Reduction or loss of Kerckring's folds + scalloped folds + mosaic pattern		
Magazzù et al, J Clin Gastroenterol (1994)	100	99
Reduction or loss of Kerckring's folds + scalloped folds + mosaic pattern+ visibility of blood vessels		
Mauriño et al, Dig Dis Sci (1993)	94	92

Endoscopy

The endoscopic appearance of the duodenum may be strongly suggestive of celiac disease. A number of endoscopic signs have been described, and the loss or reduction of duodenal folds and the scalloped configuration of reduced folds have been the endoscopic features most extensively studied (Fig. 2). Many studies agree that reduction in height and number of folds is the most evident single endoscopic change in adults, whereas its childhood counterpart is represented by the scalloping of folds, suggesting the existence of an age-dependent spectrum of endoscopic alterations in this condition. However, other endoscopic signs, such as the mosaic pattern of duodenal mucosa with visibility of the underlying vessels and a diffuse micronodular pattern in the duodenal cap, have also been described. Table 1 summarizes their sensitivity and specificity values as deduced from published studies, although some of them included only small series of celiac patients and were not performed blindly. An increase in sensitivity without a proportional reduction of specificity is evident if we look simultaneously for more than one marker.

Finally, it has been suggested that push-type enteroscopy can provide a valuable tool in the screening of celiac disease. However, since endoscopic markers, when present, are already evident in the duodenum, there is no reason to prefer more expensive equipment and procedures that are more time-consuming and require specifically trained medical staff. On the other hand, enteroscopy represents a valuable tool in the recognition of some complications of celiac disease, such as intestinal lymphoma and ulcerative jejunoileitis.

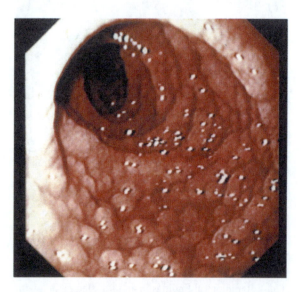

Fig. 2. Endoscopic pattern of untreated celiac disease. The presence of multiple nodularity in the duodenal cap may reveal the diagnosis of adult celiac disease

Serological test

Anti-gliadin and anti-endomysium immunoglobulins are two circulating antibodies strictly associated with celiac disease. The search for their presence in the serum is currently used as a screening test, being valuable in terms of sensitivity, specificity, and of cost-effect ratio. Their use should be particularly reserved for risk groups of celiac disease such as first-degree relatives and patients suffering from the abovementioned associated diseases.

Definitive diagnostic test

Histology

The histologic appearance of duodenal/jejunal biopsy specimens is considered the gold standard for the diagnosis of celiac disease. The characteristic lesions consist of villous atrophy, crypt hyperplasia and hypertrophy and mononuclear infiltrate both in the epithelium and in the lamina propria. These features, however, are not pathognomonic on their own, but if gliadin/prolamine withdrawal from the diet leads to their significant improvement, the diagnosis is confirmed. Even milder lesions should be considered indicative of celiac disease, providing they respond unequivocally to a gliadin-free diet. A second biopsy after one year of diet is, therefore, needed to achieve an indisputable diagnosis.

As far as the position of endoscopy in the diagnostic work-up of celiac disease is concerned, its role is negligible and may be even misleading with respect to those patients already suspected of having this condition on clinical and/or serological grounds. In this clinical setting the decision to perform biopsies must not depend on marker detection during endoscopy. On the contrary, the search for these markers may be of crucial importance during an endoscopy performed for other reasons as confirmed by the diagnosis of unsuspected new celiac patients following this policy (Figs. 3-5).

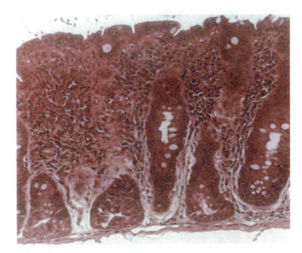

Fig. 3. Histological finding in untreated adult celiac disease. The complete absence of duodenal villi, hypertrophy and hyperplasia of crypts and chronic flogistic infiltrate in epithelium and lamina propria are evident

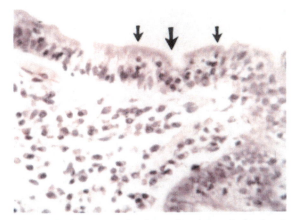

Fig. 4. Higher magnification of untreated duodenal mucos. *Arrows* point to the increased density of intraepithelial lymphocytes

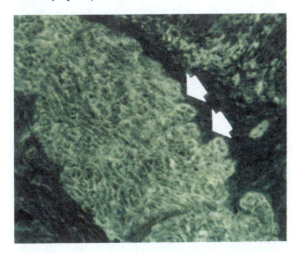

Fig. 5. *Arrows* indicate positive staining at indirect immunofluorescence in monkey esophagus endomysium after incubation with serum from a celiac patient

Suggested reading

Brocchi E, Corazza GR, Caletti G, Treggiari EA, Barbara L, Gasbarrini G (1988) Endoscopic demonstration of loss of duodenal folds in the diagnosis of celiac disease. N Engl J Med 319:741-744

Corazza GR, Gasbarrini G (1995) Coeliac disease in adults. Bailliere's Clin Gastroenterol 9:329-350

Trier JS (1991) Celiac sprue. N Engl J Med 325:1709-1719

Tropical sprue
F. Klotz

Two centuries ago tropical sprue was identified as a chronic diarrhea syndrome with malabsorption of unknown etiology that affected patients living in tropical regions or who had lived in such regions.

It is different from subclinical tropical malabsorption which has occurrence consequences. It is associated with a persistent gastrointestinal symptomatology, even after the person has left the endemic zone, and proteinocaloric-deficient pernicious anemia. It responds favorably to treatment associating antibiotics and folic acid.

Regardless of time and space, this syndrome affects both natives and travellers. The symptomatology may appear many weeks after coming back from the tropics. The syndrome can be sporadic or endemic.

The beginning of tropical sprue is usually brutal with febrile acute diarrhea, and it sometimes occurs in an epidemic context. Some patients do not recover and develop sprue.

It seems to be an infectious disease. The pathogenic agent probaby is an intestinal bacterium. Some researchers have found high concentrations of bacteria in jejunum. *Klebsiella pneumoniae, Escherichia coli, Enterobacter cloacae*, and more recently an protozoon, *Cyclospora cayetanensis*, have been incriminated.

Tropical sprue is the consequence of colonization of the small bowel. This colonization perpetuates through factors resulting in a clinical and biological syndrome. This infectious hypothesis is widely supported by the great sensitivity of this disease to antibiotics.

After the initial episode, the symptomatology becomes chronic with chronic diarrhea and the malabsorption syndrome.

Chronic evolution may sometimes result in considerable weight loss accompanied by a deterioration in the general state.

To diagnose tropical sprue we may proceed by elimination, starting with parasitosis, celiac disease, Whipple's disease, intestinal lymphoma and mycobacteriosis.

The approach is:

Clinical: The beginning of the disease is in endemic zones or on arrival home from the tropics with clinical signs of deficiency suggesting malabsorption.

Biological: We notice the presence of at least two biological syndrome elements of malabsorption (steatorrhea, perturbation of the test at the D xylose, pernicious anemia with vitamin B_{12} or folic acid deficiency).

Histological: Endoscopy does not provide objective macroscopic evidence, but makes biopsy sampling possible. Lesions start in the duodenum and the jejunum and more towards the ileum. There is partial and patchy villous atrophy with a more specific element that shows the presence of a lipid band under the coating epithelium revealed with *Soudan coloration*. That band could play a role in the malabsorption.

Radiological: Radiological images in tropical sprue are not typical for the disease; dilated loops with transversal and thick contours are possible.

Suggested reading

Cook GC (1996) Tropical sprue: some early investigators favoured an infective cause, but was a coccidian protozoan involved? Gut 39:428-429

Rambaud JC, Ngo Y (1993) Traitment des infections bactériennes chroniques de l'intestin grele, pullulations bactériennes chroniques, sprue tropicale et maladie de Whipple. Ann Gastroeneterol Hepatol 29:4:189-197

Whipple's disease

G.R. Corazza, M. Di Stefano, M.A. Pistoia

In 1907, George Whipple described the case of an adult man who died from an unknown disease characterized by the presence of a massive infiltration of small intestinal mucosa by voluminous and foamy PAS+ macrophages, mesenterial adenopathy, pleuritis, pericarditis and endocarditis. Thus, the multisystemic nature of the disease was evident, right from the original description. Only very recently has it been recognized that the disorder is due to an infection with *Tropheryma whippelii*, a gram-positive actinomycetes, perhaps precipitated by a pre-existing defect of cellular immunity. Such an infection may virtually involve all organs and tissues, thus making an impressive polymorphism in the clinical features possible.

More than 85% of all patients reported are middle-aged men. The most frequently reported symptoms are diarrhea, weight loss, arthralgia, anorexia, fever, anemia, lymphadenopathy, cutaneous hyperpigmentation. Less frequently vasculitis, porpora, arterial thrombosis, congestive heart failure, pericarditis and gastrointestinal bleeding have been reported. Involvement of the central and peripheral nervous systems are observed with increasing frequency at presentation and represent the most common site of disease relapse after treatment with drugs that do not penetrate uninflamed meninges.

Approach tests

Radiology
Radiology has no discriminating role in the diagnosis of Whipple's disease. Nonspecific radiologic features are thickened folds, flocculation and fragmentation of the barium column.

Endoscopy
The most frequent endoscopic pattern in Whipple's disease consists of the presence of a pale yellow, shaggy mucosa or whitish-yellow punctate lesions in the descending duodenum and proximal jejunum due to secondary lymphangiectasia, alternating with endoscopically normal mucosa. Friable erythematous mucosa and erosions may also be present (Figs. 1, 2).

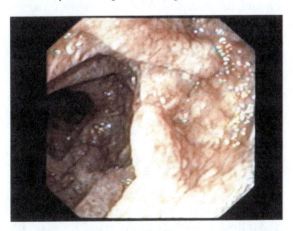

Fig. 1. Endoscopic appearance of the jejunum in a patient with Whipple's disease. Thickened folds seem to be coated with yellow-white material in a patchy distribution (by courtesy of Prof. J. Bures, Hradek Kralove, Czech Republic)

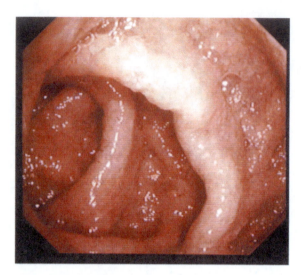

Fig. 2. Jejunal Whipple's disease (by courtesy of Prof. F.P. Rossini, Turin, Italy)

Definitive diagnostic test

Histology

The diagnosis of Whipple's disease is at present based on histological demonstration of characteristic PAS+ macrophages with foamy cytoplasm in the duodenal and jejunal lamina propria or in any other involved organ. This massive infiltrate may cause enlargement and shortening of villi, together with obstruction of the lymphatic vessel with consequent lymphangiectasia. Macrophage PAS positivity reflects the presence of glycoproteins derived from the incomplete degradation of bacterial cells within macrophage lysosomes. It should be noted that infection with *Mycobacterium avium intracellulare* in patients with AIDS is histologically similar to Whipple's disease, but can be ruled out by Ziehl-Neelsen staining, which does not identify *T. whippelii*.

Histological demonstration of characteristic PAS+ macrophages in the involved organ represents the current basis for the diagnosis of this condition. Recently, the amplification by polymerase chain reaction of a specific region of *T. whippelii* genome in various tissues and in cerebrospinal fluid has been performed. A broader application of this new test will perhaps represent an important improvement in the diagnosis and follow-up of this condition in light of recent results showing molecular detection of *T. whippelii* in biopsy samples taken from histologically negative mucosal areas.

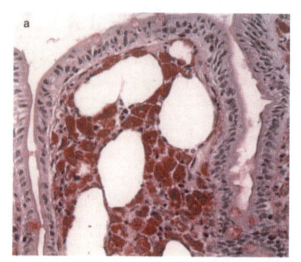

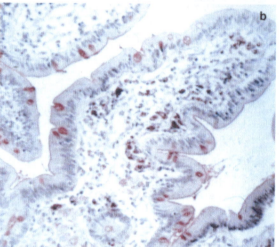

Fig. 3. a Histological appearance of mucosa in a patient with untreated Whipple's disease. Villi are enlarged and shorter than normal. Dilated lymphatics and PAS+ foamy macrophages are evident in the lamina propria (PAS; original magnification x 140). **b** Histological appearance of mucosa 1 year after antibiotic therapy. Villi appear to be less distorted, there is no evidence of lymphatic dilation, and only a few PAS+ macrophages are visible (PAS; original magnification x 140)

Suggested reading

Muller C, Peterman D, Stain C, Riemer H, Vogelsang H, Schnider P, Zeiler K, Wrba F (1997) Whipple's disease: comparison of histology with diagnosis based on polymerase chain reaction in four consecutive cases. Gut 40:425-427

Relman DA, Schmidt TM, McDermott RP, Falkow S (1992) Identification of the uncultured bacillus of Whipple's disease. N Engl J Med 327:293-301

Volpicelli NA, Salyer WR, Milligan FD, Bayless TM, Yardley JH (1976) The endoscopic appearance of the duodenum in Whipple's disease. Johns Hopkins Med J 138:19-23

Ulcerative jejunoileitis
G.R. Corazza, M. Di Stefano, M.A. Pistoia

Ulcerative jejunoileitis is a rare condition characterized by the presence of multiple and transverse ulcerations located in the jejunum, the ileum or both, with consequent scarring that can lead to narrow strictures of the intestinal wall. This condition has been considered to be a complication of adult celiac disease for 30 years, since the report of a case in which celiac disease had been diagnosed with certainty long before the development of small intestinal ulcerations. Very recently, ulcers of the first and second part of the duodenum have also been found in two very young celiac children. The nosology of this condition is today very confused. Even when coupled with villous atrophy, the dependence on celiac disease may be questionable in patients who do not respond to gluten withdrawal.

Guide symptoms

On clinical grounds, although ulcerative jejunoileitis may be very rarely asymptomatic, the mortality is very high (over 70%) due to surgical complications, such as obstructions, bleeding or perforation. Colicky central abdominal pain, abdominal distention, low-grade fever, diarrhea, weight loss and nutritional deficiencies are the most frequent symptoms and should alert physicians to this condition particularly in patients with a previous history of malabsorption or of celiac disease.

Approach tests

Radiology
Radiology, even by enteroclysis, is unreliable in showing ulcerations that are, however, indirectly suggested by the evidence of strictures in patients who complain of the above-mentioned symptoms (Fig. 1a).

Endoscopy
A valuable new tool for the direct recognition of ulcers of the proximal jejunum is push-type enteroscopy. In intestines showing thickening and inflammation, the mucosa is affected by numerous transverse fissure-type ulcerations. Strictures are responsible for dilation of the adjacent segments.

Histology
Full-thickness non-specific and non-granulomatous inflammation and various degrees of villous atrophy in adjacent mucosa are the main histological features of this condition (Fig. 1b). Granulomas are absent, denying the dependence of the above features on preexisting Crohn's disease, whereas gastric metaplasia is often found in the vicinity of the ulcers. In some cases ulcers may be associated with microscopic aggregates of neoplastic cells, suggesting that prelymphoma cells may be responsible for the enteropathy and ulceration.

Definitive diagnostic test

In the majority of the patients described to date, ulcerative jejunoileitis has been diagnosed by radiology or at laparotomy/autopsy (Fig. 1c). There is no doubt that enteroscopy, which can also be performed during laparotomy, represents a new fundamental tool for the recognition of this condition. Its dependence on preexisting celiac disease can be confidently confirmed by the positivity of anti-endomysium antibodies.

Suggested reading

Bayless TM, Kapelowitz RF, Shelley WM, Ballinger WF, Hendrix TR (1967) Intestinal ulceration – a complication of celiac disease. N Engl J Med 276:996-1002

Green JA, Barkin JS, Gregg PA, Kohen K (1993) Ulcerative jejunitis in refractory celiac disease: enteroscopic visualization. Gastrointest Endosc 39:584-585

Losowsky MS (1995) Ulcerative jejunoleitis-nosological, morphological and clinical aspects. In: Gasbarrini G, Corazza GR, Alessandrini A (eds) Morfologia dell'intestino tenue. Editrice Compositori, Bologna, pp 79-85

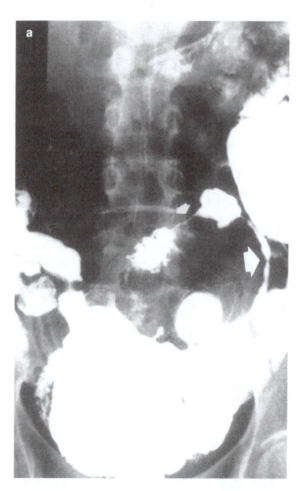
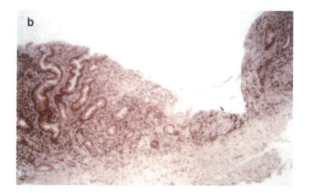
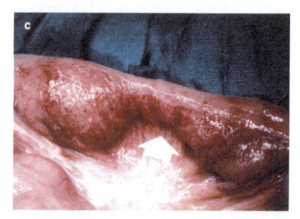

Fig. 1. a Enteroclysis in a patient with ulcerative jejunoileitis. *White arrows* show close strictures with proximal distention of the lumen. **b** Histological appearance of ulcerative jejunoileitis. An ulceration partially filled with granulation tissue (*right*) and surrounded by chronic inflammatory cell is evident in the context of villous atrophy with crypt hypertrophy (hematoxylin-eosin; original magnification x 20). **c** Laparotomy: *arrow* indicates stricture of an intestinal loop

Eosinophilic enteropathy

E. Brocchi, R. Corinaldesi

Eosinophilic enteropathy (synonyms: eosinophilic gastroenteritis, eosinophilic enteritis) is a rare disease, in which eosinophils may infiltrate different layers of the gut wall. Any area of the gastrointestinal tract can be involved, but especially the stomach and small bowel.

Although any age group can be affected, patients generally are from 20 to 50 years old, with a slight male prevalence.

In order to establish the diagnosis, the following criteria need to be fulfilled: presence of gastrointestinal symptoms, histologic demonstration of eosinophilic infiltration of one or more areas of the gastrointestinal tract, absence of parasitic infestation, absence of eosinophilic involvement of organs outside the gastrointestinal tract.

Neither food intolerance nor allergy or peripheral blood eosinophilia is required for the diagnosis, as many patients do not have any evidence of these.

The pathogenesis is poorly understood. A lot of data strongly suggest that eosinophils may directly damage the gastroenteric wall in this disease, by releasing intra/cellular granules (containing some cationic proteins) that can produce disruption of external cell membranes.

What may cause infiltration and degranulation of eosinophils with tissue damage is largely unknown: an allergic mechanism has most commonly been postulated, but only in a minority of cases have specific antigens (dietary allergens, drugs, toxin exposure) been demonstrated.

The symptoms are typically intermittent and long-standing, generally for years. Clinical and pathological forms, include mucosal, muscle and serosal layer disease; specific symptoms of the three forms are sometimes additive and overlap. The most prevalent form has predominantly mucosal and submucosal involvement, and symptoms include abdominal pain, nausea, vomiting, diarrhea, weight loss; iron-deficiency anemia, protein-losing enteropathy or malabsorption may be associated.

Patients with predominant muscle layer disease typically present with pyloric or intestinal obstruction; most often pathologic changes are localized, although rare diffuse involvements are described. Related symptoms are crampy abdominal pain, nausea and vomiting.

The rarest form is serosal layer disease; the whole bowel is often involved, and the clinical feature is eosinophilic ascites.

Diagnosis

Peripheral blood eosinophilia is found in about 80% of cases. Iron-deficiency anemia can occur, probably due to blood loss in the mucosal layer disease; serum albumin level may be low in this clinical form. Severe protein loss can also result in low immunoglobulin levels. The serum IgE level may be elevated, particularly in children. In order to rule out parasitic infestation, stool studies need to be obtained in all cases. Stools may be positive for occult blood. Mild-to-moderate steatorrhea is present in up to 30% of cases.

Radiologic studies

Variable and non-specific X-ray changes may be found in this disease; in at least 40% of cases X-ray films may be normal. Gastric folds can be enlarged with mucosal involvement and nodular filling defects. In muscle layer disease, there may be localized involvement of the antrum and pylorus, causing narrowing and gastric retention. Thickening of the folds with or without nodules may be found in mucosal small bowel disease; narrowing of some areas with dilation of proximal tracts can be seen in muscle layer involvement. Echo tomography and computed tomography may demonstrate thickened intestinal walls and sometimes localized mesenteric lymphadenopathy; with serosal involvement, ascitic fluid usually is detected.

Endoscopy and histology

Endoscopic findings may vary from a normal mucosa to prominent folds, hyperemia, erosions, ulcerations or nodularity. The patchy involvement of the gastrointestinal tract in this disease strongly suggests that multiple biopsies should be obtained by enteroscopy from the stomach and upper small bowel, both from normal and from abnormal areas. Histologic evaluation of samples represents the best way to make a firm diagnosis. Edema and infiammatory cell infiltrate (almost entirely composed of eosinophilis) involving the gut wall are the predominant findings of this disease; necrosis and regeneration of the surface and glandular epithelium may also be found. It must be underlined that a significant increase in other inflammatory cells makes the diagnosis of eosinophilic gastroenteritis unlikely. If eosinophilic gastroenteritis is suspected, patients with previous histologically normal samples should have repeat biopsies. In patients with muscle layer disease, mucosal biopsies are often not conclusive; full-thickness samples may thus be required, although surgery should be avoided if clinical, laboratory and radiologic findings make eosinophilic gastroenteritis highly likely.

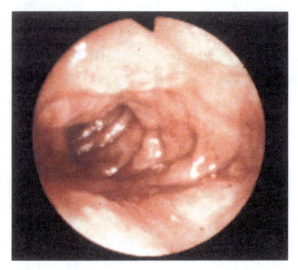

Fig. 1. Endoscopic picture showing edema, hyperemia and thickening of jejunal folds

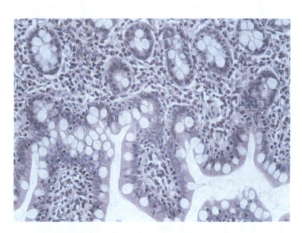

Fig. 2. Endoscopic biopsy of the jejunum showing a large number of eosinophils within the mucosa (courtesy of Prof. W. Grigioni, Bologna, Italy)

Suggested reading

Cello JP (1979) Eosinophilic gastroenteritis: a complex disease entity. Am J Med 67:1097-1101

Talley NJ, Shorter RG, Phillips SF, Zinsmeister AR (1990) Eosinophilic gastroenteritis: a clinicopathological study of patients with disease of the mucosae, muscle layer and subserosal tissues. Gut 31:54-57

Vitellas KM, Bennett WF, Bova JG, Johnson JC, Greenson JK, Caldwell JH (1995) Radiographic manifestations of eosinophilic gastroenteritis. Abdom Imaging 20:406-413

Vasculitis

G. Gay, J.S. Delmotte

Vasculitis is a multisystem disorder characterized by the inflammation and necrosis of blood vessels and is classified by the size of the affected vessels. Organs with the richest vascular supply such as the gastrointestinal tract are often affected.

Strong evidence supports the concept that vasculitis manifested as a leukocytoclastic process is linked to immune complex disease with immune-circulating complex deposit and abnormal cell-mediated immune response in the wall of the arteries with consequent inflammation and necrosis of the involved tissues.

Gastrointestinal involvement in vasculitis is marked by aneurysm medium-sized arteries that can rupture and bleed massively (PAN). Vasculitis of small arteries provokes segmental ischemia ulcerations and occult bleeding (Henoch-Schönlein purpura) (Table 1).

Table 1. Classification of vasculitis * (modified from Desbazeille F, Soule JC, 1986)

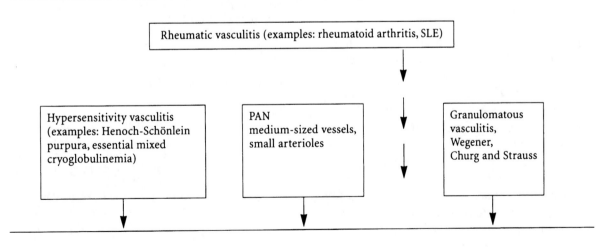

* Gastrointestinal location of larger-vessel vasculitis such as giant cell arteritis are not mentioned because this is rare

Involvement of the small intestine

Polyarteritis nodosa (PAN) involves small to medium arteries. Gastrointestinal symptoms include abdominal pain and diarrhea, which are present in two-thirds of cases. Vascular occlusions lead to ischemia with mucosa ulcerations that provoke gastrointestinal bleeding. Drugs such as corticosteroid and cyclophosphamide increase the bleeding risk of these ulcerations.

In Henoch-Schönlein purpura – small-size vasculitis – the percentage of gastrointestinal symptoms varies from 29% to 69%. Bleeding is common in relation to segmental ischemia and ulcerations.

Rare in Wegener's granulomatosis, ulcerations with upper and lower-bleeding are common in patients with systemic lupus erythematosis (SLE).

Radiology

In Henoch-Schölein, a small-bowel enema shows a decrease in peristalsis, a thumb print in the margin, and little nodules in the jejunum. Echotomography and CT scan demonstrate the consequences of ischemia: absence of lumen and thickness of the wall of the small bowel.

Enteroscopy

One should remember that enteroscopy should be performed with caution without excess insufflation in patients with vasculitis.

It is useful when gastrointestinal symptoms appear during treatment to distinguish the specific symptoms of vasculitis from drug-associated gastrointestinal lesions.

Enteroscopy may be useful for the diagnosis. Two cases of HBV-related PAN with severe, extensive duodenal and jejunal ulcerations have been reported. Extensive serpiginous and aphthous ulcerations were present in the second part of the duodenum. In these two observations, active PAN were found on the biopsies. In Henoch-Schönlein purpura, enteroscopy demonstrates multiple jejunal nodules, erythema and ulcerations.

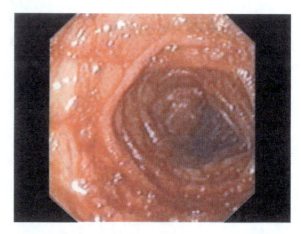

Fig. 1. Multiple jejunal ulcerations in a patient with active bleeding. Biopsy specimen: vasculitis

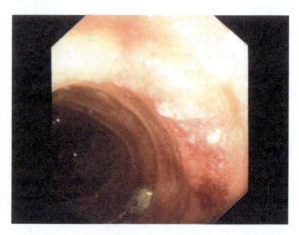

Fig. 2. Jejunal lesion characterized by hyperemia, edema and ulceration with peripheral micronodulia in a patient with occult bleeding. Biopsy specimen: vasculitis (by courtesy of Dr. F.P. Rossini, Turin, Italy)

Suggested reading

Desbazeille F, Soule JC (1986) Manifestation digestives des vascularites. Gastroenterol Clin Biol 10:405-414

Guillevin L, Lhote F, Gallais V, Jarousse B, Royer I, Gayraud M, Benichou J (1995) Gastrointestinal tract involvement in polyarteritis nodosa and Churg-Strauss syndromes. Ann Med Interne 146:260-267

Williams DH, Kratka DC, Bonafede JP, Katon RM (1992) Polyarteritis nodosa of the gastrointestinal tract with endoscopically documented duodenal and jejunal ulcerations. Gastrointest Endosc 38:501-563

Crohn's disease

A. Arrigoni, M. Pennazio, F.P. Rossini

Crohn's disease is a chronic inflammatory disease whose etiology and pathogenesis remain unknown. It may involve the entire gastrointestinal tract, although small bowel and colon account for 98%. More than two-thirds of the cases involve the terminal ileum, and in 10%-20% other areas of the small bowel are also affected. The incidence in Western countries is 2-4 newly diagnosed cases/100,000 inhabitants/year, and the prevalence is 30-50 patients with Crohn's disease/100,000 inhabitants. While the peak occurrence is between the ages of 15 and 35 years, it has been reported in every decade of life. A familial incidence has been recorded with estimates that 2% to 5% of patients with Crohn's disease will have one or more relatives affected.

Crohn's disease is characterized by chronic inflammation extending through all layers of the intestinal wall. The disease is discontinuous, and severely involved segments are separated from each other with segments of normal bowel. At an early stage the involved bowel tract appears hyperemic and edematous. As the disease progresses, the bowel appears thickened with the lumen narrowed; mucosal ulceration may deepen into the submucosa and muscolaris and form intramural fissures or fistulas, which may occur between adherent loops or other organs.

The major clinical features of Crohn's disease are crampy abdominal pain, diffuse or localized in the right lower quadrant, diarrhea, fever and weight loss. The diarrhea is often moderate, usually without gross blood. In some patients the first manifestation may be intestinal obstruction, which is a frequent complication also in the course of the disease, occurring in 20%-30% of patients. The course of Crohn's disease is unpredictable, but it is typically characterized by alternate phases of exacerbation and remissions and by the almost inevitable recurrence of surgical interventions. Intestinal bleeding leading to sideropenic anemia can in some cases be the sole symptom and could induce in-depth diagnostic investigations.

Approach tests

Radiology
The plain film of the abdomen may demonstrate dilated bowel loops or air-fluid levels when obstruction is present. Enteroclysis is a well-established diagnostic method, not only for detecting the disease, but also for its anatomical distribution and for identifying complications.

Computed tomography (CT)
In Crohn's disease CT imaging of the abdomen may be of value in the evaluation of thickened, separated bowel loops and in helping distinguish thickened, matted loops from intra-abdominal absces.

Nuclear imaging
Radionuclide scanning techniques can be used to assess the extent of active bowel inflammation in Crohn's disease in selected patients.

Ultrasonography

Ultrasonography and color Doppler ultrasonography are effective in the evaluation of patients with small bowel Crohn's disease as increased thickness and loss of the regular stratification pattern of the bowel wall can be accurately imaged. It is a useful diagnostic tool in preliminary evaluation of patients with abdominal pain and suspected Crohn's disease.

Endoscopy

Endoscopy offers the opportunity to explore the terminal ileum with retrograde ileoscopy at the end of a total colonoscopy, the jejunum with push enteroscopy and, theoretically, the entire small bowel with sonde enteroscopy.

A variety of abnormalities of the mucosal surface can be identified: patchy erythema with focal edema, aphthous lesions, focal linear deep ulcerations, serpiginous, confluent or non-confluent ulcerations, cobblestone pattern, stenosis. The possibility to perform targeted biopsies during retrograde ileoscopy or push enteroscopy allows the diagnostic work-up to be complete in the majority of cases and, above all, a differential diagnosis to distinguish it from other pathologies can be obtained.

Indications for enteroscopy in patients with Crohn's disease

- Occult bleeding in general and, in particular, in cases of suspected Crohn's disease
- To evaluate doubtful radiologic findings and/or to confirm images indicative of Crohn's disease
- To carry out biopsies and thus to make a differential diagnosis between Crohn's disease and other diseases (IPSID, lymphoma, ulcerative jejunitis)
- To evaluate surgical anastomoses
- For precancerous screening of the small bowel
- To evaluate modifications induced by therapy

Definitive tests

When small bowel Crohn's disease is suspected, a definitive diagnosis is usually obtained by the radiological appearance at enteroclysis; histological confirmation is often possible by push enteroscopy or by retrograde ileoscopy (Table 1).

Table 1. Crohn's disease of the small bowel: recommended investigations

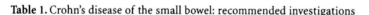

Suggested reading

Lescut D, Vanco D, Bonniere P, Lecomte-Houcke M, Quandalle P, Wurtz A, Colombel JF, Delmotte JS, Paris JC, Cortot A (1993) Perioperative endoscopy of the whole small bowel in Crohn's disease. Gut 34:647-649

Rhodes J, Mayberry JF, Roberts GM, Williams GT, Dew MJ, Harries AD (1994) Clinical features of Crohn's disease. In: Misiewicz JJ, Punder RE, Venables CW (eds) Diseases of the gut and pancreas. Blackwell Science, Oxford, pp 717-740

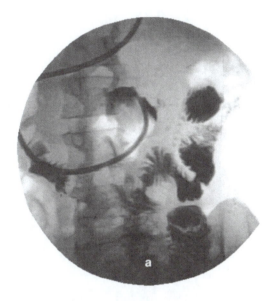

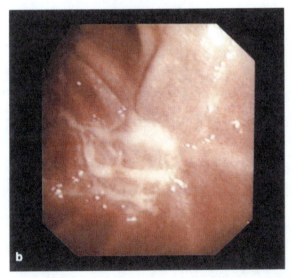

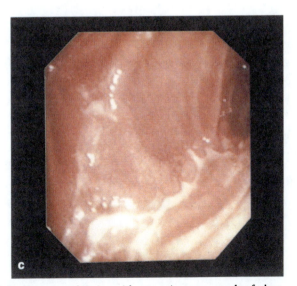

Fig. 1. a *Enteroclysis*: concentric and eccentric stenosis beyond the ligament of Treitz, with retraction as a result of ulcer healing (by courtesy of Dr. E. Juliani, Turin, Italy). *Push enteroscopy*: **b** sharply demarcated and **c** serpiginous jejunal ulcers in Crohn's disease

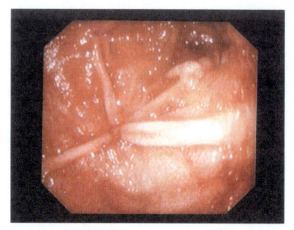
Fig. 2. Ulcer with mucosal retraction in the distal jejunum

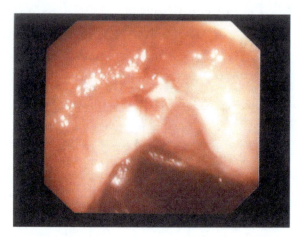
Fig. 3. Jejunal ulcer

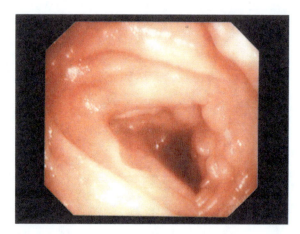
Fig. 4. Jejunal cobblestone appearance in Crohn's disease

Atlas of Enteroscopy

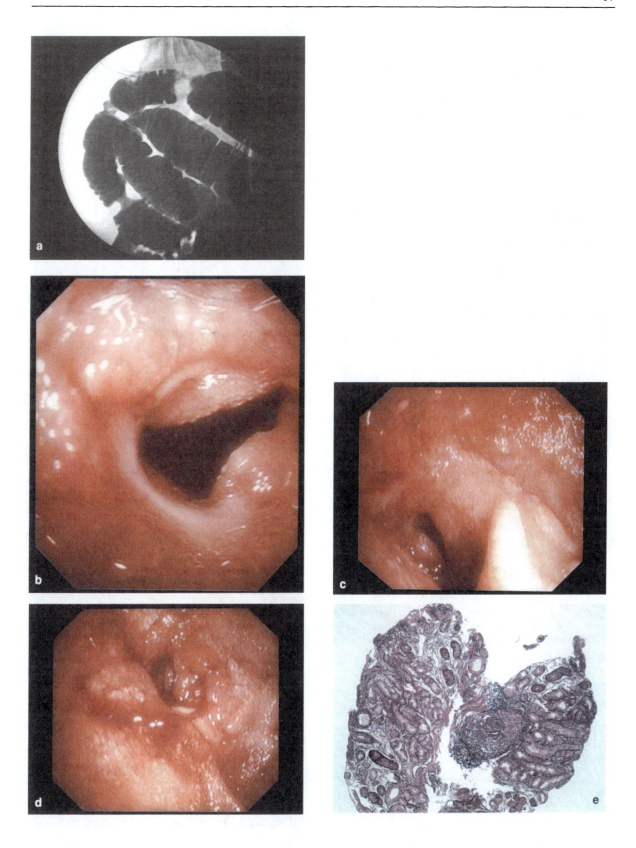

Fig. 5. a *Enteroclysis*: multiple jejunoileal stenoses (by courtesy of Dr. E. Juliani, Turin, Italy). *Push enteroscopy evaluation of the radiologic finding*: **b, c** Jejunal lumen is distorted by a fibrotic pad; the mucosa is hyperemic and edematous, with ulcerations; **d** Distal jejunal stenosis lined by hyperemic, edematous, apparently infiltrated mucosa, with small ulcers; **e** Histological examination of biopsy specimens: Crohn's disease (by courtesy of Prof. G. Palestro, Turin, Italy)

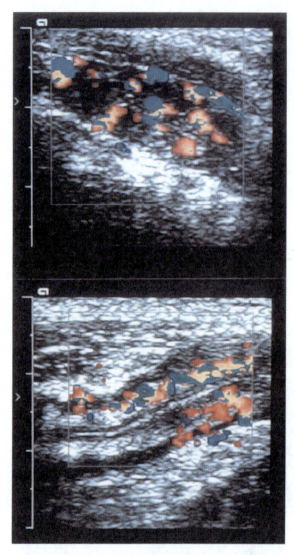

Fig. 6. Color Doppler ultrasonography of a thickened bowel loop in a case of active Crohn's disease. The bowel wall is filled with color signal, arising from dilated arterial and venous vessels typical of inflammation-related hyperemia (by courtesy of Prof. L. Bolondi, Bologna, Italy)

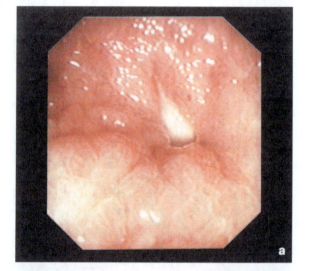

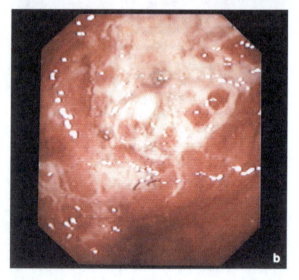

Fig. 7. a Anastomotic stenosis in a recurrence of jejunal Crohn's disease. **b** Endoscopic evaluation after therapy: a large ulceration surrounding punctiform stenosis of jejunoileal anastomosis is shown

Amyloidosis

G. Gay, J.S. Delmotte

Amyloidosis is characterized by the infiltration of tissues by amyloid proteins. Gastrointestinal involvement is common in all types of amyloidosis.

Biochemical studies show four different types of amyloid proteins: amyloid A with protein (AA) in secondary amyloidosis; right chain protein (AL) in primary or myeloma-associated amyloidosis; prealbumin (AF) in various types of familial amyloidosis; and two microglobulin (AH) in hemodialysis amyloidosis. Deposits of amyloid substance in the lamina propria mucosae result in malabsorption diarrhea and mucosal friability with occult bleeding. A deposit in muscular mucosae explains impaired intestinal motility.

Whatever the type, amyloidosis produces a clinical presentation in relation to the organ infiltrated: kidney, brain, heart, muscle, liver, spleen, pancreas, tongue salivary glands and jaws. A high occurrence of amyloid deposits in the small intestine has been reported, one-third of the cases at necropsy. Small intestine involvement often reveals the disease: dyspepsia, diarrhea/constipation at the beginning of the disease, then malabsorption, exudative enteropathy, and bleeding complicate the evolution.

In gastrointestinal involvement the diagnosis is performed with biopsy specimens of the jejunum by enteroscopy. Examination of the specimen stained with congo red under polarized light shows the presence of green deposits. Chemical types of amyloid proteins are identified by specific antibodies in the biopsy specimen.

Endoscopy

When the small intestine is involved, an abnormal appearance is observed endoscopically in two-thirds of the patients. A fine granular appearance is present in 60% of patients, erosions and mucosal friability in 43%, thickening of the valvulae in 20%, multiple yellowish-white polypoid protusions in 17% and shallow ulcers in 10%. A fine granular appearance may be characteristic of AA amyloidosis (Fig. 1a).

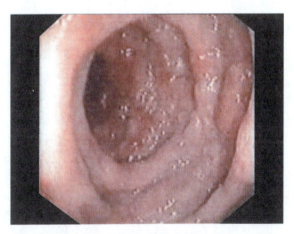

Fig. 1.a Thickening of jejunal folds with granular nodular appearance

Intestinal endoscopy is useful when amyloidosis is suspected, especially if gastrointestinal manifestations are present. The appearance endoscopically characteristic, especially if yellowish infiltration of the thick valvulae is present. A definitive diagnosis can be obtained with intestinal biopsy specimens, and the type of amyloidosis can then also be determined (Fig. 1b).

Suggested reading

Gay G, Delmotte JS (1996) What use for the enteroscopy. Gastroenterol Clin Biol 20:B127-B133

Gillat T, Revac H, Sohaur E (1969) Deposition of amyloidosis in the gastrointestinal tract. Gut 10:98-104

Tada S, Lida M, Yao T, Kawakubo K, Okada M, Fujishima M (1994) Endoscopic features in amyloidosis of the small intestine: clinical and morphologic differences between chemical types of amyloid proteins. Gastrointest Endosc 40:45-50

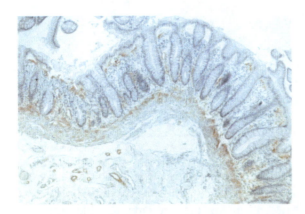

Fig. 1.b Biopsy specimen: AA amyloidosis (by courtesy of Dr Y. Grignon, Nancy, France)

Sarcoidosis

G. Gay, J.S. Delmotte

Sarcoidosis is a systemic disorder of unknown cause. The non-caseating granuloma is the characteristic feature. The disease is self-limited with a favorable course or chronic with episodic recrudescence and remissions.

Even though the cause of sarcoidosis remains obscure, geographical, immune, genetic and infectious factors are suspected to play a crucial role. Also the development of sarcoidosis implies: exposure to antigens, acquired cellular immunity directed against the antigen, overexuberant cellular immune response. The role of T-cell lymphocytes is important for antigen recognition and amplifications of the local cellular immune response. The granuloma is the consequence of this acute and chronic inflammation in the organ involved.

The clinical manifestations of sarcoidosis are protean. It involves only one organ or several at the same time. Usually systemic symptoms are present: fatigue, anorexia, weight lost and fever. More acute presentations are associated with erythema nodosum, bilateral hilar lymphoadenopathy, polyarthralgies known as Lofgren's syndrome.

There is respiratory tract involvement in the course of the disease in nearly all cases of sarcoidosis, but digestive localization is rare. Liver localization is usual, and one-third of patients have hepatomegaly or a cholestatic profile of biochemical alterations. Diarrhea and exudative enteropathy are the clinical expression of gastrointestinal localization, especially if there is disseminated gastrointestinal sarcoidosis. However, several publications suggest that a subclinical inflammation of the gut is present in active pulmonary sarcoidosis.

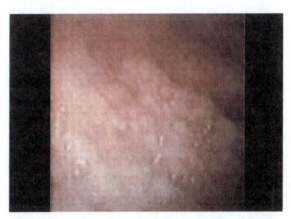

Fig. 1. Disseminated nodular aspect of the jejunal mucosa

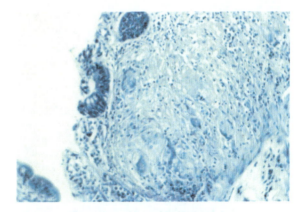

Fig. 2. *Sarcoidosis*: granuloma with giant cells

The endoscopic appearance of the mucosa may be nodular or normal even if the disease is disseminated along the jejunum. Biopsy specimens are demonstrative of the granuloma (Figs. 1, 2).

Diagnostic procedure

The endoscopic aspect is not suggestive. Nodules are common in other diseases, such as lymphoma. The diagnosis is suspected if pulmonary lesions are known. In their absence, biopsy specimen of the nodular lesion will confirm sarcoidosis.

Suggested reading

Godeau B, Farcet JP, Delchier JC, Xuan DH, Chaumette MT, Gaulard P (1992) Proteins losing enteropathy in gastrointestinal sarcoidosis associated with malignant lymphoma. J Clin Gastroenterol 14:78-80

Newman LS, Rose CS, Maier LA (1997) Sarcoidosis. N Engl J Med 336:1224-1234

Wallaert B, Colombel JF, Adenis A, Manchandise X, Hollgren R, Janin A, Tonnel AB (1992) Increased intestinal permeability in active pulmonary sarcoidosis. Am Rev Respir Dis 145:1440-1445

Mastocytosis

G. Gay, J.S. Delmotte

Mastocytosis is an overproliferation and accumulation of tissue mast cells. Mast cell disease is most commonly seen in the skin, and it occurs in adults more than children. Other organs that are involved are the skeleton, bone marrow, central nervous system and the gastrointestinal tract.

Mast cells are distributed in every organ close to blood and lymphatic vessels, peripheral nerves and epithelial surfaces. Mast cells play a main role in inflammatory functions. The reason why mast cells proliferate and accumulate in various organs is unknown.

Five distinct diseases are identified according to the classification of Golkar:

- Cutaneous mastocytosis
- Systemic mastocytosis with or without skin involvement
- Mastocytosis with hematological disorder
- Lymphadenopathic mastocystosis
- Mast-cell leukemia

The skin is most commonly involved, but this is not obligatory. Gastrointestinal symptoms are numerous and common in systemic mastocytosis: epigastric pain, lower abdominal discomfort, watery diarrhea malabsorption, steatorrhea. Exudative enteropathy is often seen as well as peptic disease with complications.

Enteroscopy

Segmental nodular lesions of 2-5 mm are characteristic, disseminated on flat jejunal mucosa. This aspect is also present in the stomach and the duodenum.

Diagnostic procedure

When cutaneous lesions are present, the diagnosis is confirmed by skin biopsy. In unclear cases, or in the absence of skin lesions, bone marrow biopsy and biopsies from different organs involved should be made in order to demonstrate the excess and infiltration of mast cells.

If clinical suspicion
- Clinical and histological examination of skin
- Complete blood count
- Histamine, prostaglandine urine tests
- 24-h urine collection mediators to exclude other disorders
- Bone marrow biopsy and aspiration

Staging
- Bone and abdominal scan
- Upper endoscopy and enteroscopy
- Encephalic MRI

Suggested reading

Golkar L, Bernhard JD (1997) Mastocytosis. Lancet 349:1379-1385

(Figs. 1, 3, 4 by courtesy of Drs. Meier and Bischoff, Hannover, Germany)

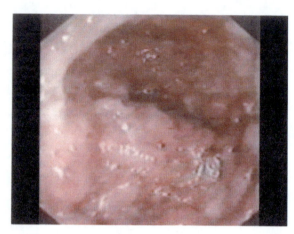

Fig. 2. Jejunal nodular lesions

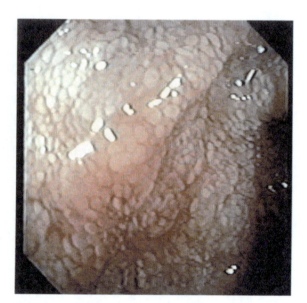

Fig. 3. Branlike pattern of the jejunal mucosa

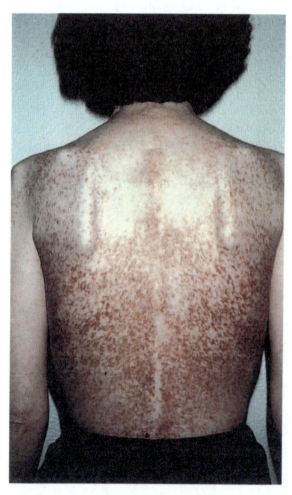

Fig. 1. Skin lesions due to mastocytosis

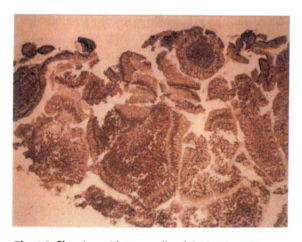

Fig. 4. Infiltration with mast cells of the lamina propria

Abeta and hypobetalipoproteinemias

G. Gay, J.S. Delmotte

Abetalipoproteinemia (ABL) and hypobetalipoproteinemia (HBL) are a heterogeneous group of genetic disorders. They have in common low, indetectable levels of plasma Apo-B or Apo-B containing lipoproteins: chylomicrons, very low density lipoproteins (VLDL) and light density lipoproteins (LDL). In plasma they are characterized by undetectable or low plasma triglyceride and cholesterol.

Abetalipoproteinemia is a rare – 100 patients reported – autosomal, recessive disease. The genetic defect is in the assembly and secretion of VLDL in the liver and of the chylomicrons in the intestine in the absence of microsomal tryglyceride transfer proteins (MTP), resulting in retinitis pigmentosa, spinocerebellar degeneration with ataxia, fat diarrhea, malabsorption syndrome of fat-soluble vitamins.

Hypobetalipoproteinemia is an autosomal dominant disorder caused by a mutation or deletion in the apoB gene which produces a truncated Apo B. Plasma concentrations of the two forms of apolipoprotein B, that is, Apo B-100 synthetized by the liver and Apo-B48 synthetized by the intestine, are undetectable. The biological and clinical pictures are similar to those in abetalipoproteinemia. Heterozygote HBL disease is present in 0.1%-0.8% of the general population. Homozygote HBL is rare whereas the prognosis of those two Apo B related disorders mainly depends on the consequences of the malabsorption syndrome and on the progressive neurological alterations caused by a deficiency in soluble vitamin E.

Diagnostic procedure

In peripheral blood examinations: hypocholesterolemia, acanthocytosis, undetectable Apo-B lipoprotein.

Enteroclysis
This procedure exhibits dilation of the jejunum and the ileum with thick mucosa in relation to the fat infiltration of the small intestine.

Enteroscopy
This procedure demonstrates snowy and yellow coloration of the small intestine without atrophy all along the small intestine.

CT scan
This procedure shows a massive and diffuse infiltration of the liver.

Histopathology
Liver: massive steatosis and mitochondrial alterations are seen. Small intestine (jejunum and ileum) shows accumulation of fat vacuoles within biopsies of the enterocytes, no villous atrophy.

Immunohistochemistry
- Migration of truncated Apo-B and absence of normal Apo-B hypobetaliproteinemia for hypobetalipoproteinemia
- Absence of migration of Apo-B and truncated Apo-B for abetalipoproteinemia

Suggested reading

Gay G, Pessah M, Bouma ME, Roche JF, Aymard JP, Beucler I, Aggerbeck LP, Infante R (1990) L'hypobetalipoproteinémie familiale. Etude familiale de 4 cas. Rev Med Interne 11:273-279

Scoazec JG, Bouma ME, Roche JF, Blache D, Verthier N, Feldmann G, Gay G (1992) Liver fibrosis in a patient with familial homozygous hypobetaliproteinemia: possible role of vitamin supplementation. Gut 33:414-417

Wetterau JR, Aggerbeck LP, Bouma ME, Eisenberg C, Munck A, Hermier, Schmitz J, Gay G, Rader DJ, Gregg RE (1992) Absence of microcosmal tryglyceride transfer proteins in individuals with abetalipoproteinemia. Science 258: 99-1001

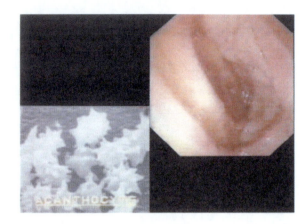

Fig. 1. c *Top right*: yellow fat infiltration of the jejunal folds; *bottom left*: acanthocytosis

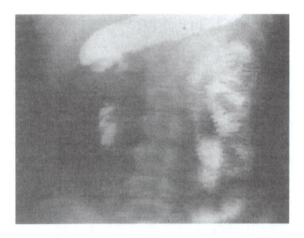

Fig. 1. a Enteroclysis: massive infiltration and thickening of jejunal folds

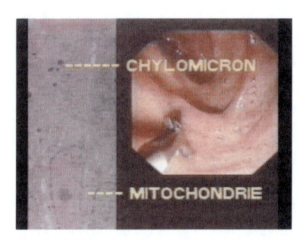

Fig. 1. d Enteroscopic jejunal biopsy: excess chylomicrons in the mitochondria (EM)

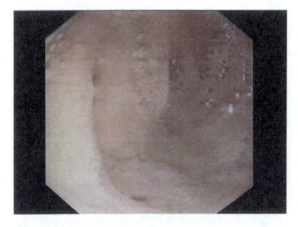

Fig. 1. b Enteroscopy: yellow and snowy appearance of the normal mucosa

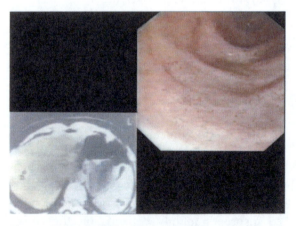

Fig. 1. e *Top right*: diffuse fatty infiltration in the ileum; *bottom left*: liver steatosis (CT scan)

Hypogammaglobulinemia

G. Gay, J.S. Delmotte

Hypogammaglobulinemia disorders are categorized into two groups: (1) secondary to leukemias, lymphomas, host graft disease and (2) primary. The last group is considered here.

In adults common variable hypogammaglobulinemia and selective IgA deficiency are the most frequent.

Primary hypogammaglobulinemia may be congenital or acquired. The defect in these disorders has not been identified, although in the majority of cases there appears to be a specific metabolic defect or a disorder of gene regulation. The consequences are: defects in the cellular components of the immune system or a decrease in their secretory products.

Table 1. Selective IgA deficiency: clinical manifestations

GASTROINTESTINAL	EXTRAINTESTINAL
• Infections • Gluten-sensitive enteropathy (IgA prevalence is 1: 50) • Pernicious anemia • Rare nodular lymphoid hyperplasia • Crohn's disease (prevalence is 1: 73)	• Collagen vascular disease • Atopy • Risk of malignancy is rare

(Modified from Targan and Shanahan)

Table 2. Common variable hypogammaglobulinemia: clinical manifestations

GASTROINTESTINAL	EXTRAINTESTINAL
• *Giardia lamblia* infection • Small bowel bacterial overgrowth • Viral and infectious diarrhea • Gluten-sensitive sprue and refractory sprue • Frequent nodular lymphoid hyperplasia, not premalignant	• Recurrent respiratory tract infection • Increase risk of lymphomas • Increase risk of gastric cancer

(Modified from Targan and Shanahan)

Enteroscopy

Nodular changes of the mucosa predominate in the jejunum, but the totality of the small bowel may be involved. There is neither dilation nor fold thickening. If an infection is superimposed, congestive and inflammatory folds are seen in the jejunum. Endoscopic appearances suggesting villous atrophy are identifiable if gardiasis and/or gluten enteropathy is present

Microscopically, the nodules consist of large follicles with germinal centers within the lamina propria; plasma cells are absent. This aspect is different from the localized form of nodular lymphoid hyperplasia, which may occur in immunocompetent children in the terminal ileum.

From a practical point of view, enteroscopy is useful to obtain biopsy specimens from nodular lymphoid hyperplasia, to prove intestinal infection (lambliasis) or to search for villous atrophy when enteropathy refractory to a gluten-free diet is suspected.

Suggested reading

Teahon K, Webster AD, Price AB, Weston J, Bjarnason I (1994) Studies on the enteropathy associated with primary hypogammaglobulinemia. Gut 35:1244-1249

Targan SR, Shanahan F (1992) Gastrointestinal manifestations of immunologic disorders in: Textbook of gastroenterology (vol 2). In: Yamada T (ed) Lippincott, Philadelphia, pp 2455-2471

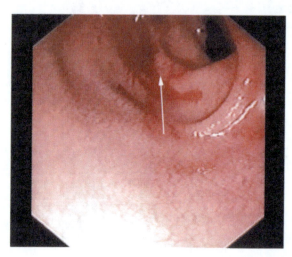

Fig. 1. A biopsy performed on a small nodule surrounded by atrophic jejunal mucosa

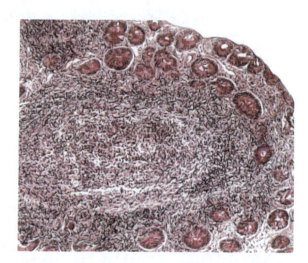

Fig. 2. *Ig A deficiency*: follicular hyperplasia with absence of plasma cells (by courtesy of Dr. Y. Grignon, Nancy)

TUMORS

Small bowel tumors

Primary gastrointestinal lymphoma

Carcinoid tumors of the small bowel

Small bowel tumors

F.P. Rossini, M. Risio

Tumors of the small bowel represent about 5% of all primary neoplasms of the gastrointestinal tract. The incidence is probably underestimated, diagnostic methods not being very effective, in particular when the neoplasm, whether benign or malignant, is small in size.

Even if most small bowel tumors originate within the intestinal wall, at a relatively early phase their expansive infiltrative growth produces an alteration in the endoluminal surface. This makes endoscopic identification possible, followed by biopsy sampling and histopathological evaluation, if required.

Nevertheless, only rarely, above all in tumors of stromal origin, can endoscopic biopsy afford the full definition of the histotype. The specimen only provides a generalized histogenesis (vascular, stromal, lymphoid) of the lesion.

Small bowel tumors, whether primary or metastatic, benign or malignant, cause intermittent abdominal pain, episodes of occlusion, weight loss, nausea, and vomiting. The most important clinical finding indicating a neoplasia of the small bowel, in particular in patients below the age of 50 years, is occult bleeding with secondary iron-deficiency anemia.

In these cases, after having excluded pathologies responsible for bleeding in the upper gastrointestinal tract, all diagnostic effort should be aimed at the small bowel.

There are numerous diagnostic tests to approach this particular pathology: small bowel follow-through or enteroclysis is certainly the first investigation, followed by CT scan and angiography.

Push enteroscopy can identify tumors, including small ones, in the jejunum; in theory, sonde enteroscopy can do the same throughout the entire small bowel.

It is very difficult to define an algorithm; the sequence of the various procedures must always be correlated to the clinical picture and be dictated by rational indications.

Table 1. Classification of small bowel tumours

EPITHELIAL TUMORS
Benign:
- Adenoma
- Adenomatosis (FAP)

Malignant:
- Adenocarcinoma

NON-EPITHELIAL TUMORS
- Lipoma
- Vascular tumors (hemangioma - lymphangioma - Kaposi sarcoma)
- Gastrointestinal stromal tumours (GIST)
  - With smooth muscle differentiation (leiomyoma, leiomyosarcoma, leiomyoblastoma)
  - With neural differentiation (schwannoma, plexosarcoma, gastrointestinal autonomic nerve tumors (GANT)
  - Uncommitted type
- Neurofibroma and neurofibromatosis
- Gangliocytic paraganglioma
- Ganglioneuroma and ganglioneuromatosis
- Paraganglioma

TUMOR-LIKE LESIONS
- Hamartoma:
  - Peutz-Jeghers polyp and polyposis
  - Juvenile polyp and polyposis
- Heterotopias (pancreatic - gastric)
- Hyperplasia of Brunner's glands
- Inflammatory fibroid polyp
- Canada-Cronkite polyposis
- Lymphoid hyperplasia
- Benign lymphoid polyp and polyposis
- Lipohyperplasia of ileocecal junction
- Endometriosis

METASTATIC TUMORS

MALIGNANT LYMPHOMAS
B-cell:
- Lymphomas of mucosa-associated lymphoid tissue (MALT):
  - Low-grade and high-grade B-cell lymphomas of MALT
  - Immunoproliferative small intestinal disease (IPSID)
- Mantle-cell-type lymphoma (lymphomatous polyposis)
- Burkitt-like lymphoma
- Low-grade and high-grade lymphomas corresponding to lymph node equivalents

T-cell:
- Enteropathy-associated T-cell lymphoma (EATL)
- Other T-cell lymphomas

ENDOCRINE TUMORS
- Carcinoid tumors

Adenoma

Adenomatous polyps may be found in the small bowel. The most frequent location is the duodenum or jejunum, with the diameter varying from a few millimeters to several centimeters, sessile or pedunculated.

Although radiology is the primary method, endoscopic identification and removal is the definitive diagnostic test, in particular for prevention of carcinoma.

Small bowel adenomas are essentially similar to those of the large bowel, although the villous or tubulovillous architecture is prevalent in the small bowel, perhaps in relation to the normal villous anatomy of the mucosa in this segment. The premalignant potential of small bowel adenomas is reliably attested, and histological evidence indicates malignant transformation of adenomatous tissue during the early phases. Thus, an adenoma-carcinoma sequence may reasonably be considered in the genesis of small-bowel carcinoma. Colonic metaplasia and progressive ingravescence of dysplasia are assumed to be the initial alterations of the epithelium.

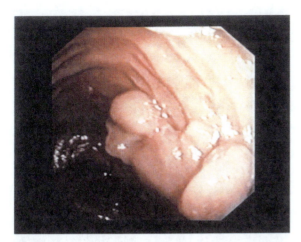

Fig. 1. Ulcerated sessile adenomatous polyp of the jejunum

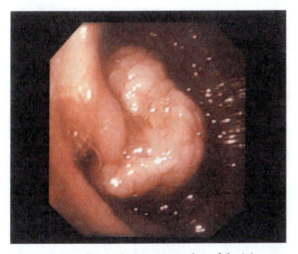

Fig. 2. Pedunculated adenomatous polyp of the jejunum

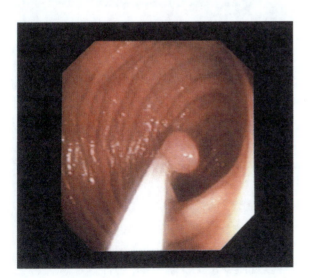

Fig. 3. Endoscopic polypectomy of an adenoma

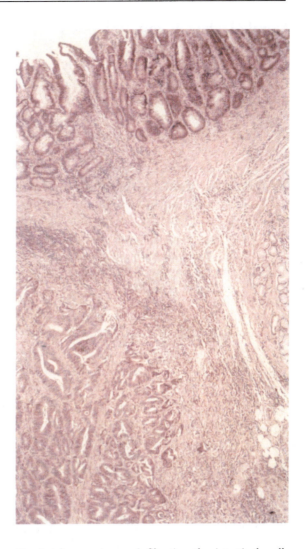

Fig. 4. Adenocarcinoma infiltrating the intestinal wall, originating from the adenomatous tissue with high-grade dysplasia, which has entirely replaced the mucosa lining

Familial adenomatous polyposis (FAP)

In FAP, cancer of the upper digestive tract is the most frequent cause of death, after proctocolectomy; the incidence of adenomas, precursors of carcinoma, is particularly significant in the duodenum, in the periampullar region and in the jejunum. Thus, in FAP, identification and removal of adenomas are highly advisable for the prevention of cancer. The adenomas being mainly located in the duodenum and proximal jejunum, push enteroscopy might thus be sufficient to complete surveillance of the digestive tract; with the side-viewing duodenoscope, evaluation of the papilla of Vater and of the surrounding region is guaranteed.

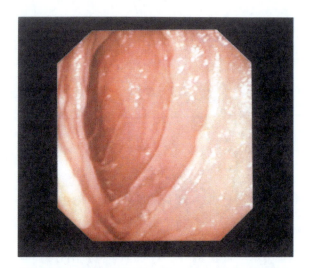

Fig. 1. Numerous small jejunal prominences in FAP. Histological finding of adenoma

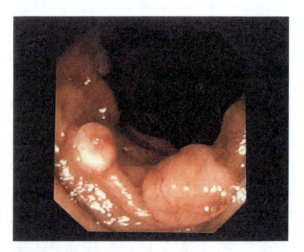

Fig. 2. Sessile adenoma in FAP

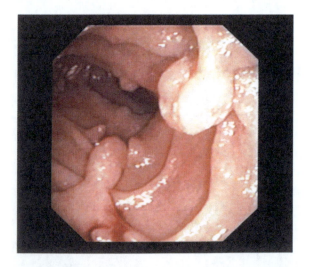

Fig. 3. Multiple adenomas of variable morphology in FAP (by courtesy of Prof. J. Bures, Hradek-Kralove, Czech Republic)

Adenocarcinoma

Most adenocarcinomas of the small bowel are located in the duodenum and proximal jejunum and thus may be diagnosed by push enteroscopy. The diagnostic approach is in general radiological.

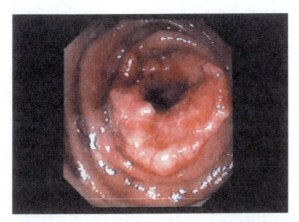

Fig. 1. a *Push enteroscopy*: vegetation with wide base, ulcerated, stenotic, in the jejunum in a patient with occult bleeding

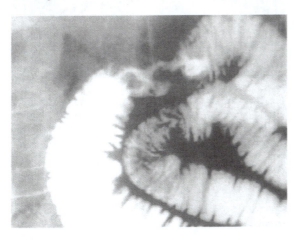

Fig. 1. b *Enteroclysis*: rapid evolution of the neoplasia induces stenosis of the bowel. Typical characteristics are narrowing and rigidity of the lumen, eccentric passage of the contrast medium, ulceration, and slow peristalsis

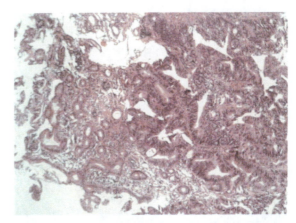

Fig. 1. c Histologic characteristics are similar to those observed in adenocarcinomas of the large bowel, although in the small bowel the incidence of anaplastic forms is higher. Various different histotypes (mucinous adenocarcinoma, signet ring cell carcinoma, adenosquamous carcinoma, mixed glandular-endocrine cell carcinoma) have been identified. Since small-bowel adenocarcinoma originates via the sequence adenoma-carcinoma, and in 80% of resected carcinomas there are residues of adenomatous tissue, multiple targeted biopsies should be performed for correct diagnosis of the tumor

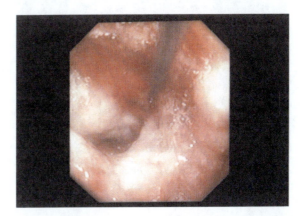

Fig. 2. Infiltrating stenotic adenocarcinoma of the jejunum

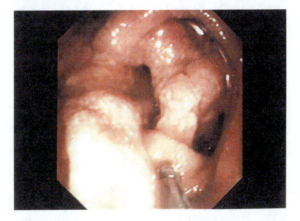

Fig. 3. Vegetating adenocarcinoma of the jejunum (by courtesy of Prof. G. Gay, Nancy, France)

Hemangioma

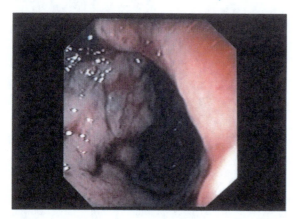

Fig. 1. a *Cavernous hemangioma.* Swollen bluish extramucosal formation, with nodular surface, soft, elastic consistency when probed with biopsy forceps, bleeding upon slight pressure from biopsy forceps

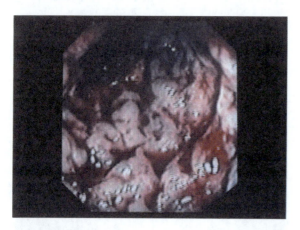

Fig. 1. b *Diffused cavernous hemangioma.* Multiple bluish areas, high probability of bleeding, involving an extensive section of the jejunal lumen

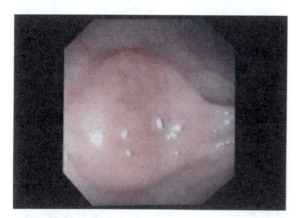

Fig. 1. c *Nodular hemangioma.* Swollen, polypoid formation with wide base, with central umbilication covered with seemingly regular mucosa, regular, soft elastic consistency (by courtesy of Profs. M. Ingrosso and A. Francavilla, Bari, Italy)

Neurofibroma and neurofibromatosis

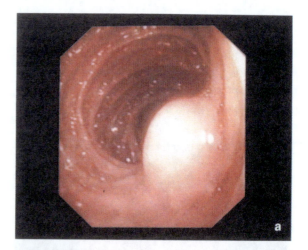

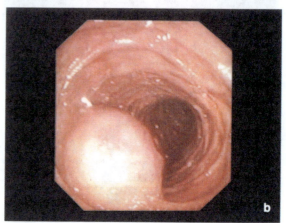

Fig. 1. a, b *Push enteroscopy*: multiple nodules of hard elastic consistency, covered with smooth mucosa, mobile on the underlying plane, located in the jejunum; they may be related to neurofibroma in patients with cutaneous neurofibromatosis. Some nodules may show ulceration responsible for bleeding. Endoscopic biopsy is not generally diagnostic.

Leiomyoma

These are among the most frequently found small bowel tumors. In 80% of cases they are located in the jejunum ileum, in 20% of cases in the duodenum.

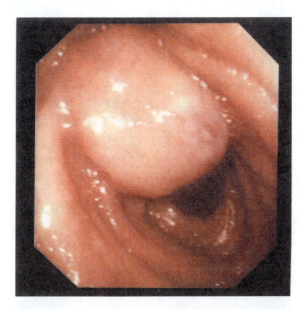

Fig. 1. *Push enteroscopy*: at the distal jejunum, a submucosal formation is detected, with a wide base, non-mobile on the underlying plane, coated with smooth, pink mucosa and a hard, elastic consistency. Ulcerated umbilication is clearly visible, with bleeding edges responsible for occult bleeding. Endoscopic biopsy is not determinant

Leiomyosarcoma

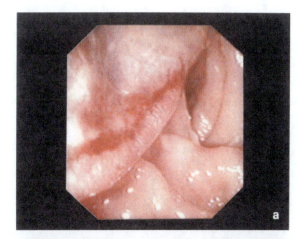

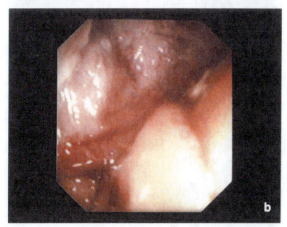

Fig. 1. a, b *Push enteroscopy*: the lumen of the distal jejunum is deformed, substenotic, impeding further insertion of the instrument. Infiltration and rigidity of the folds are clearly visible, delimiting large areas of necrosis. Histological finding at endoscopic biopsies: leiomyosarcoma

Small bowel tumors

Gastrointestinal autonomic nerve tumors (GANT)

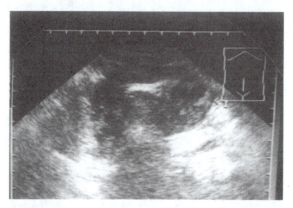

Fig. 1. a *Ultrasonography*: typical kidney-shaped aspect indicating a solid tumor

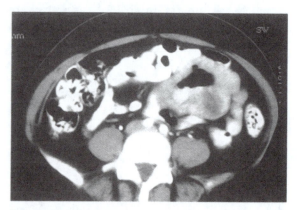

Fig. 1. b *CT scan*: excavated tumor with asymmetrical thick walls and regular polycyclical shape without fibrous infiltration and no mechanical consequences

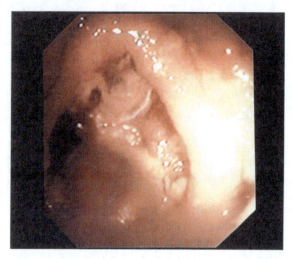

Fig. 1. c *Push enteroscopy*: large scar-lobe-shaped polypoid stenotic tumor with central ulceration

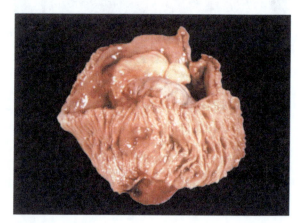

Fig. 1. d Surgically resected intestinal segment histology - GANT tumor

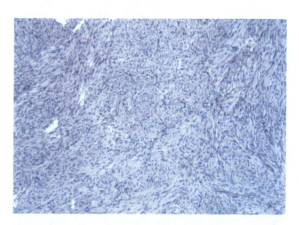

Fig. 1. e Spindle cells arranged in interlaced bundles. Neoplastic cells show elongated, mostly blunt-ended nuclei (by courtesy of Profs. G. Gay and D. Regent, Nancy, France)

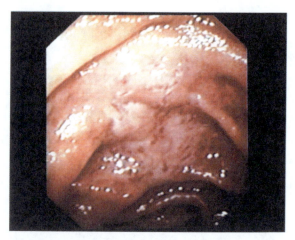

Fig. 2. *Push enteroscopy*: a different endoscopic appearance of the mucosa (vascularlike lesion) in GANT tumor of the jejunum (by courtesy of Dr. A. Van Gossum, Brussels, Belgium)

Peutz-Jeghers' polyp and polyposis

Peutz-Jeghers polyps are generally multiple, pedunculated, with a wide base, and varying from a few millimeters to 4-5 cm.

As well as being found in the large bowel and the upper stretch of the gastrointestinal tract, a high percentage is found in the small bowel.

Enteroclysis is a very important test and is determinant both for diagnosis and for the definition of the therapeutic strategy, since it affords a map of the location of the polyps. The polyps are exported by endoscopy and/or surgery. This strategy can result in complications, such as intussusception, occlusion and bleeding (Figs. 1-5).

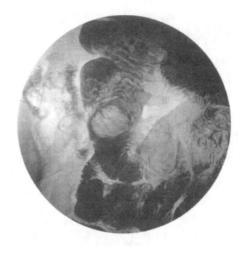

Fig. 1. a *Enteroclysis*: a large polyp of the jejunum

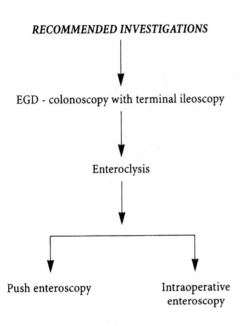

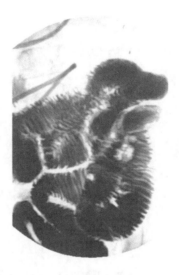

Fig. 1. b *Enteroclysis*: multiple small jejunal polyps

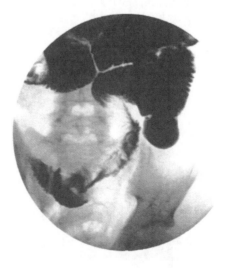

Fig. 1. c *Enteroclysis*: Jejunoileal intussusception
(Fig. 1a-c by courtesy of Dr. E. Juliani, Turin, Italy)

RECOMMENDED INVESTIGATIONS

↓

EGD - colonoscopy with terminal ileoscopy

↓

Enteroclysis

↓

Push enteroscopy   Intraoperative enteroscopy

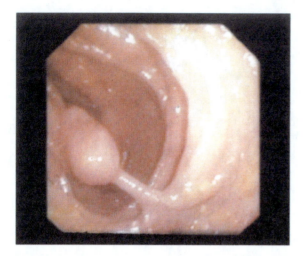

Fig. 2. *Push enteroscopy.* Pedunculated polyp of the jejunum

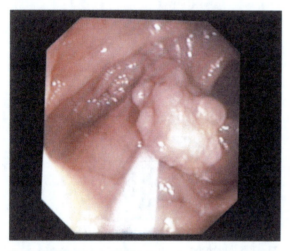

Fig. 3. *Push enteroscopy.* Endoscopic polypectomy of a sessile polyp of the jejunum

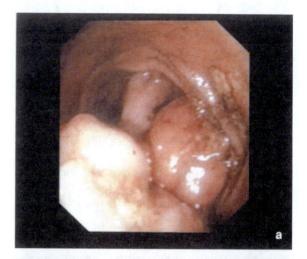

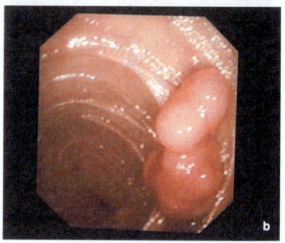

Fig. 4. a, b *Intraoperative enteroscopy.* Large sessile and pedunculated polyps of the ileum

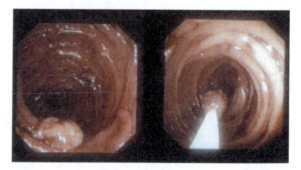

Fig. 5. *Intraoperative enteroscopy.* Endoscopic polypectomy during intraoperative enteroscopy

Metastatic tumors

Metastatic tumors can occur in the small bowel and can sometimes simulate a primary tumor.

Metastatic tumors may on occasion be found by chance during an investigation to identify the location and nature of occult bleeding. The tumors that can most frequently metastastize in the ileal jejunum are those originating in the lungs, ovaries or stomach. The melanoma may frequently be responsible for metastasis in the various segments of the small bowel.

Suggested reading

Arrigoni A, Pennazio M, Rossini FP, (1996) Enteroscopy in small bowel neoplastic pathology. Acta Endosc 26:255-261

Jass JR, Sobin LH, (1989) Histological typing of intestinal tumours, 2 edn. Springer, Berlin Heidelberg New York

Lewis BS, Kornbluth A, Waye JD (1991) Small bowel tumors: yield of enteroscopy. Gut 32:763-765

Pennazio M, Arrigoni A, Rossini FP, (1995) Push enteroscopy for small bowel tumours. Gastrointest Endosc 41:524-525

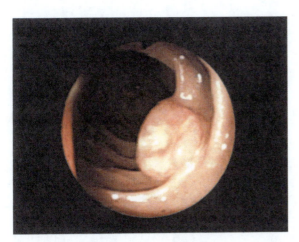

Fig. 1. Jejunal metastasis from melanoma

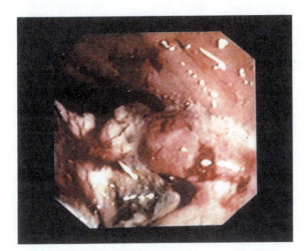

Fig. 2. Jejunal localization secondary to melanoma (by courtesy of Prof. J. Bures, Hradec Kralove, Czech Republic)

Primary gastrointestinal lymphoma

G. Gay, J.S. Delmotte

Lymphomas account for 1%-4% of all primary gastrointestinal tumors. Primary gastrointestinal lymphoma is defined as a localized or regional intestinal lymphoma in a patient with no palpable lymph nodes, no radiographic evidence of mediastinal involvement and a normal peripheral blood smear. The small intestine, especially the ileum, is involved in 21% of cases, whereas the stomach is involved in 61%.

Classification and pathogenesis of malignant lymphomas

B CELL

- Lymphomas of mucosa – associated lymphoid tissue (MALT):
  - Low-grade and high-grade B cell lymphomas of MALT
  - Immunoproliferative small intestinal disease (IPSID)
- Mantle-cell-type lymphoma (lymphomatous polyposis)
- Burkitt-like lymphoma
- Low-grade and high-grade lymphomas corresponding to lymph-node equivalents

T CELL

- Enteropathy-associated T cell lymphoma (EATL)
- Other T-cell lymphomas

Clinical presentation

Patients with Western lymphomas are usually younger than 10 years or older than 50 years. Abdominal pain is predominant.

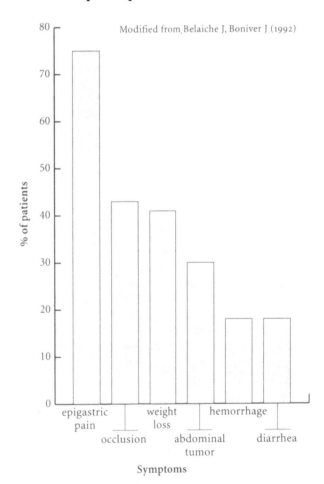

In patients with prexisting celiac disease, Western T-lymphomas should be suspected if there is a relapse despite compliance with a gluten-free diet.

IPSID is present earlier than Western lymphomas, in the second or third decade. Diarrhea is the predominant symptom. Initially, it is watery, but later it changes to steatorrhea.

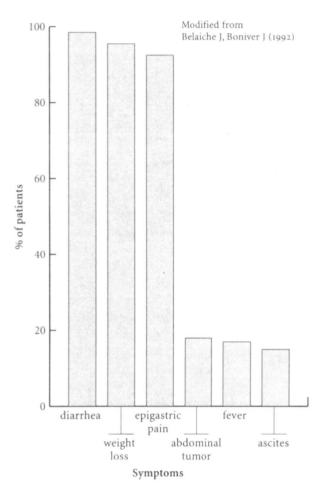

even results in intussusception, and ulcerations of mucosal lymphoma may result in considerable excavations. CT scan demonstrates thickening of the wall of the small bowel and exophytic mass. The length of abnormal small intestine is restricted in the case of Western lymphoma and very extensive in IPSID.

Push enteroscopy is useful in IPSID, as lesions are extensive and it is easier to obtain biopsies in the jejunum or in the ileum. It increases the value of endoscopic diagnosis already performed with the classic fiber upper endoscope. The endoscopic aspect shows thick folds and small nodular formation along the mucosa.

In Western lymphomas push enteroscopy is less useful than in IPSID because lesions are segmental and sometimes not accessible by push enteroscopy. When possible, inulcerative masses or polyps of different sizes, a biopsy may be made, especially lymphomatous polyposis, which is characterized by the presence of multiple lymphomatous polyps along the gastrointestinal tract. In fact, surgical exploration is necessary in numerous cases, above all in difficult situations such as suspicion of Crohn's disease or tuberculosis.

In ulcerative jejunoileitis or complicated celiac disease, T-lymphoma may develop in some patients. In suspected individuals, it is possible to obtain specific biopsies with push enteroscopy.

In the survey of long-standing celiac disease or increased lymphoma risk, as in nodular lymphocytic hyperplasia, periodic enteroscopy is mandatory to make biopsies for any suspected lesions.

Usefulness of the enteroscopy

Diagnostic steps

In IPSID, paraprotein is detectable in the peripheral blood and jejunal juice in 20% to 69%; there is no characteristic biological feature in Western lymphoma. In these conditions a few investigastions are crucial:

Barium studies demonstrate nodular imprints in the barium column because these diseases arise in the lymphoid patches. Some areas show larger polypoid lesions, which may

Suggested reading

Belaiche J, Boniver J (1992) Lymphome primitif de l'intestin grele in Gastroenterologie. (ed) Mignon M. edition Marketing / Ellipses, Paris, pp 513-524

Rambaud JC, Seligman M, Brouet JC (1994) Alpha chain disease and related lymphoproliferative disorders. In: Intestinal immunology. Ogra P. (ed) Academic Press, New York, pp 425-433

Ruskone-Fourmestraux A, Delmer A, Lavergne A, Molina T, Brousse N, Audoin J, Rambaud JC, Groupe d'Etude des Lymphomes Digestifs (1997) Multiple lymphatous polyposis of the gastrointestinal tract: prospective clinicopathologic study of 31 cases. Gastroenterology 112:7-16

Atlas of Enteroscopy

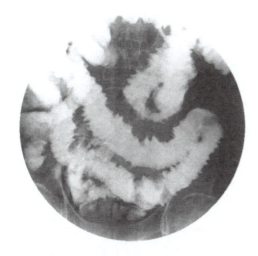

Fig. 1. *Enteroclysis*: diffuse thickening of the jejunal folds with nodularity and multiple ulcerations (by courtesy of Dr. E. Juliani, Turin, Italy)

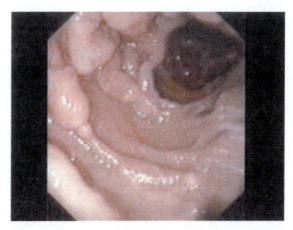

Fig. 2. *Enteroscopy*: micro- and macronodular jejunal primary lymphoma with lymphatic stasis

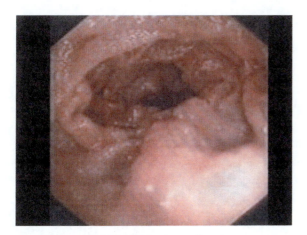

Fig. 3. Macronodular jejunal primary lymphoma

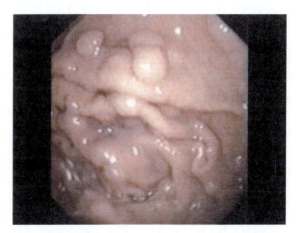

Fig. 4. Multiple lymphomatous polyposis in the jejunum

Carcinoid tumors of the small bowel

G. Delle Fave, S. Angeletti

Carcinoid tumors can be defined as neoplasms of the diffuse endocrine system which are either benign or have a more favorable prognosis than carcinomas. The characteristics are: (1) typical growth pattern (trabecular or gyriform, medullary or insular, glandular, mixture of these three types, and undifferentiated); (2) silver affinity; (3) expression of neuroendocrine markers; (4) expression of gut/brain peptides and amines.

Williams and Sanders originally proposed classifying carcinoids according to their site of origin, and this classification is useful because carcinoid tumors from these different areas differ in terms of functional manifestations, histochemistry, and secretory products (Table 1).

Carcinoid tumors can be ubiquitous, but most originate in four sites: bronchus, appendix, rectum, and jejunoileum. Overall, in the series of 8,305 cases recently published, about 74% of all carcinoid tumors occur in the gastrointestinal tract. In the gastrointestinal tract most carcinoid tumors occur in the small bowel (28.51% of total), with the highest frequency in the ileum (15.4%). The distribution of carcinoid tumors found in various surgical or clinical series differs markedly from that found at autopsy. At autopsy as many as 76% of all carcinoid tumors are found in the jejunoileum, whereas these make up approximately one-fourth of cases in clinical and surgical series. It is thus likely that a significant percentage of carcinoid tumors remain asymptomatic and undetected during life.

Small bowel carcinoids are the most frequently occurring type of carcinoid tumors. They were the second-most-frequent neoplasm encountered in the small intestine after adenocarcinoma. In the SEER (Surveillance, Epidemiology, and End Results: program of the National

Table 1. Classification of carcinoids

Origin	Organ	Immunohistochemical pattern	Clinical symptoms
Foregut	Respiratory tract	Mainly serotonin; pituitary hormones and neuropeptides	Carcinoid syndrome*
	Stomach	Gastrointestinal peptides	Flushing, gastric
	Duodenum	Serotonin, histamine	hypersecretion, diarrhea
	Jejunum		diabetes, Cushing
Midgut	Ileum	Mainly serotonin; peptides	Carcinoid syndrome*
	Appendix	of the tachynin group	None
	Right colon		Carcinoid syndrome*
Hindgut	Left colon		None
	Rectum	Multiple gut peptides	None

* Symptomatic only in cases with widespread metastases (mostly liver metastases)

Cancer Institute of the U.S.A.) files carcinoids comprised 38.6% of all small intestinal tumors. It is of interest to note that the relative frequency of small intestinal carcinoids increases in the aboral direction whereas adenocarcinomas occur in the duodenum and decrease in the aboral direction. Recent data give an annual incidence rate of 0.28:100,000 population. Also in this site, the incidence of small bowel carcinoids at autopsy is vastly greater than the clinical incidence.

Small bowel carcinoids may be multiple and 87% present within the ileum and 40% within 2 feet of the ileocecal valve. Primary tumors tend to remain small. They may spread to local lymph nodes, and a marked fibrotic reaction can occur, which distorts the gut or mesentery and can present clinically with small bowel obstruction or venous mesenteric infarction. Further spread generally occurs to the liver and possibly bone. Only approximately 20%-35% of small intestinal carcinoids are malignant and metastasize. Approximately 35% of patients with ileal carcinoid have more than one lesion (some had >100 lesions), giving the small bowel a "cobblestone" appearance. The incidence of metastases from small intestinal carcinoid tumors is dependent on the size of the primary lesion (Fig. 1).

However, the tendency for the smaller carcinoids to metastasize seems greater when the primary is in the small bowel than when it is in the rectum or appendix. In contrast to jejunoileal carcinoids, no duodenal carcinoid less than 1 cm metastasized, whereas 33% of tumors more than 2 cm or 35% of tumors invading the muscularis mucosa metastasized.

Clinical features

The presentation of small bowel carcinoid tumors that do not cause the carcinoid syndrome is related to the site of origin as well as the malignant spread of the tumor. In the appendix, carcinoid tumors are almost always found accidentally during surgery for suspected appendicitis. Small intestinal carcinoids in the jejunoileum are the most common location for carcinoid tumors of clinical significance. Most small intestinal carcinoids do not cause symptoms, but these tumors can cause fibrosis of the mesentery, which results in kinking of the bowel, intestinal obstruction, gut infarction or intussusception. The most common clinical presentation for small intestinal carcinoid is periodic abdominal pain, and intermittent crisis of

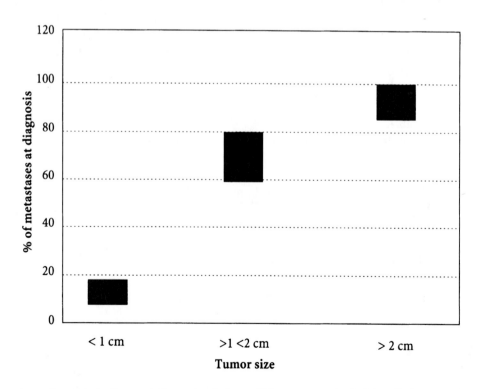

Fig. 1. Percentage of metastatic disease at diagnosis relative to different tumor size in jejunoileal carcinoids

small bowel obstruction. Because of the vagueness of the symptoms, the diagnosis of small intestinal carcinoid is frequently delayed, with the median time of onset from symptoms to diagnosis approximately 2 years, with a range of up to 20 years. Duodenal carcinoids are usually found incidentally during endoscopy. Gastrointestinal bleeding is uncommon, and these lesions are only rarely found to be ulcerated.

Diagnosis

Diagnosis of the carcinoid syndrome (characterized by flushing of the face, diarrhea, and asthma) relies on the measurement of serotonin or its metabolites (5-HIAA) in the urine. 5-HIAA determinations alone have a 73% sensitivity and a 100% specificity for the carcinoid syndrome. Some recent studies have demonstrated the increased sensitivity of measuring platelet serotonin levels, with respect to urinary 5-HIAA levels. Furthermore, also the Chromoganin-A represents a serum marker, used for diagnosis of neuroendocrine tumors; in carcinoid tumors the sensitivity is more than 80%.

A number of techniques including endoscopy, gastrointestinal barium radiographs, imaging studies (ultrasound, computer tomography (CT) scan, magnetic resonance imaging, angiography) endoscopic ultrasound, and somatostatin receptor scintigraphy (SRS) have all been used to detect tumoral lesions as well as tumor extent (Figs. 2, 3, 4a, 4b).

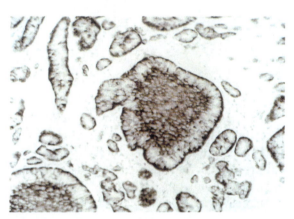

Fig. 2. *Typical carcinoid of the ileum*: characteristic argentaffine positivity (EC cells) (by courtesy of Prof. C. Bordi, Parma, Italy)

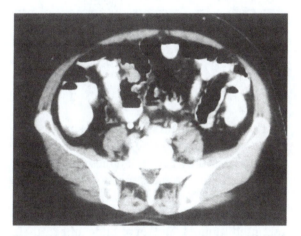

Fig. 3. Magnetic resonance imaging in a patient with ileal carcinoid (polipoid lesion jutting within the intestinal loop)

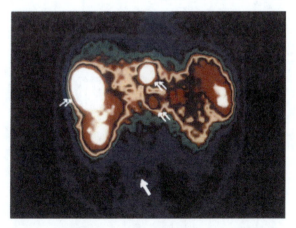

Fig. 4. a Pre-surgery somatostatin receptor scintigraphy (Octreoscan) in patient with ileal carcinoid (*one arrow*), and multiple hot spots in the liver (*double arrow*: metastases)

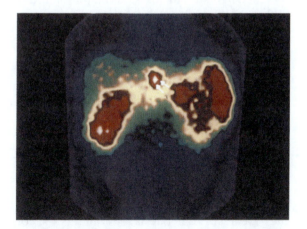

Fig. 4. b The same patient as in Fig. 4a, after debulking surgery. Only one remaining hot spot in the liver was present (*double arrow*)

Table 2. Sensitivity of somatostatin receptor scintigraphy in primary or metastatic carcinoid tumor sites

Report	No. of patients	Tumor	Sensitivity (%)
Krenning et al. (Eur J Nucl Med 1993)	37	P	86
Weinel et al. (Ann Surg 1993)	3	P	100
Kwekkebom et al. (Eur J Nucl Med 1993)	76	M	60
Lamberts et al. (Endocr Rev 1991)	39	PM	95
Van Dongen et al. (Eur J Nucl Med 1992)	4	PM	100
Scillaci et al. (J Nucl Med 1996)	18	PM	90

P = Primary; M = Metastatic

Table 3: Five-year survival (%) of carcinoid tumors of the foregut, midgut, and hindgut by stage

	Localized	Regional	Distant
Foregut	70.8-84	40-70.1	11.7-21.5
Midgut	67.6-85.4	54.4-75.2	25.2-34.8
Hindgut	70.7-81.1	44.4-46.8	18.3-20.5

The main problem is localizing small bowel carcinoids, which may be very small and frequently missed by barium studies. Virtually all (90%) carcinoid tumors possess functioning somatostatin receptors. Interaction with these receptors is the mechanism by which SRS image carcinoid tumors and octreotide affect their biologic activity. The sensitivity of SRS is very high (about 90%) and the difference in results obtained in many studies is less than 10%. Today SRS is the best single imaging technique to identify the presence, location and extent of carcinoid tumors (Table 2).

Twenty-five percent of small bowel carcinoids are localized and do not have metastases at the time of diagnosis. The presence of metastatic disease at the time of diagnosis is of 39% and 31% for locoregional and for distant metastases, respectively. The presence of regional and distant metastases (as might be predicted) is associated with a significant worsening in prognosis (Table 3). For small bowel carcinoids the 5-year survival rate is 65% and 35.9% for localized tumors and tumors with distant metastases, respectively.

The cure rate for small bowel carcinoids is exceedingly high for patients with disease localized in the small bowel. However, in patients with resectable regional nodal metastases, after 25 years of follow-up, only 23% of patients were recurrence-free.

Suggested reading

Jensen RT, Norton JA (1997) Carcinoid tumors and the carcinoid syndrome. In: De Vita V, Helman S, Rosenberg SA (eds) Cancer: principles and practice of oncology, 5th edn, pp 1704-1723

Modlin IM, Sandor A (1997) An analysis of 8305 cases of carcinoid tumors. Cancer 79:813-829

Schillaci O, Scopinaro F, Angeletti S, Tavolaro R, Danieli R, Annibale B, Gualdi G, Delle Fave G (1996) SPECT improves the accuracy of somatostatin receptor scintigraphy in abdominal carcinoid tumors. J Nucl Med 37:1452-1456

Williams ED, Sanders M (1963) The classification of carcinoid tumors. Lancet 1:238-239

OTHER INDICATIONS

Enteroscopy and AIDS

Enteroscopy of the transplanted small bowel

Uncommon endoscopic appearances of the small bowel mucosa

Enteroscopy and AIDS

Ch. Florent

The majority of AIDS patients exhibit gastrointestinal symptoms at some time during the course of their illness. These symptoms are related to pathogens or neoplasms of the gastrointestinal tract.

At the time of initial infection by HIV, patients may complain of odynophagia or, less commonly, dysphagia. Endoscopy demonstrates giant, well-defined ulcerations of the esophagus.

During the course of the illness, most patients experienced diarrhea and abdominal pain. The small intestine is involved in most cases. Enteroscopy may be useful in some cases for diagnosis. In other cases, e.g., cytomegalovirus infections, enteroscopy is not useful because of colonic and/or gastric lesions.

Kaposi's sarcoma (KS)

KS is the most common AIDS-related tumor. At least one-third of AIDS patients have KS. The incidence of KS is highest in homosexual AIDS patients. Cutaneous KS usually precedes the development of gastrointestinal and multinodal disease. Visceral involvement is found in more than 50% of cases. Any or all portions of the gastrointestinal tract may be involved. The most frequent site of involvment of the GI tract is the duodenum.

Radiology

Early flat lesions are not commonly demonstrated on barium studies, even using the double-contrast technique. As KS lesions coalesce, they enlarge and become more nodular. Smooth submucosal nodules with or without central umbilication are typical for KS.

Endoscopy

KS lesions typically appear as violescent macules or nodules measuring 5-15 mm. Endoscopic biopsy has a low yield owing to the submucosal location of the tumor. Only 25% of endoscopic biopsy specimens of KS lesions are positive in clinical practice. Pharyngeal and prepyloric lesions are very common, and multiple lesions (oropharynx esophagus, stomach and duodenum) are observed in most cases. Histological confirmation is not mandatory, except before radiotherapy or chemotherapy (Figs. 1-3).

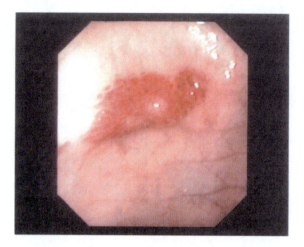

Fig. 1. Early lesion of typical Kaposi's sarcoma of the small intestine

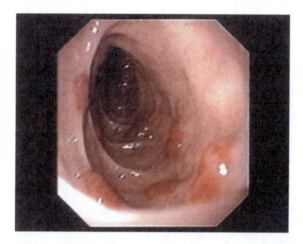

Fig. 2. Kaposi's sarcoma of the distal duodenum, multiple prominent nodules

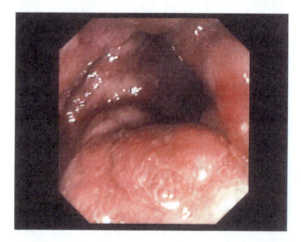

Fig. 3. Extensive, coalescent Kaposi's lesions of the small intestine

Mycobacterium avium intracellular (MAC) infections of the small bowel (pseudo-Whipple's disease)

MAC infections of the GI tract are very common in AIDS. MAC are the most common opportunistic pathogen at postmortem in patients with AIDS. The pathophysiology and anatomic aspects are similar to Whipple's disease.

Clinical enteritis is characterized by diarrhea with occult blood loss. Bacteremia involving MAC produces a wide array of clinical symptoms, including wasting, fever, night sweats, and malaise.

Radiology

Abdominal computed tomography usually shows hepatosplenomegaly and peritoneal and retroperitoneral lymphadenopathies of very low density. Barium studies, when performed, show mild small bowel dilation and diffuse, irregular fold thickening.

Endoscopy

The lesions extend from the duodenum to the distal ileum. The villi appear coarse, lymphatic stagnation gives the mucosa a milky white appearance, and the intensity of the alteration is uniform. Biopsies must be performed for histology and culture.

Histology

Pathologic examination of biopies shows infiltration with foamy histiocytes containing abundant acid-fast bacilli within expanded intestinal villi, with no mucosal exudation or ulceration. Electron microscopy may be used to confirm the localization of bacteria in macrophages (Figs. 4a-d).

Atlas of Enteroscopy

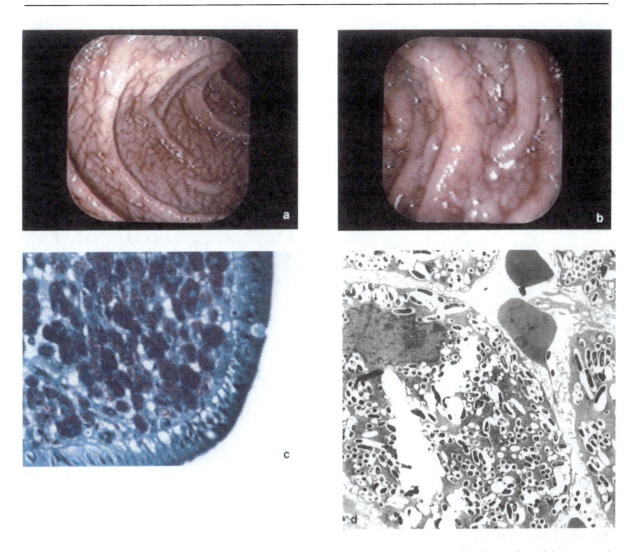

Fig. 4. a Jejunal aspect of mycobacterium avium complex of the jejunum, mimicking Whipple's disease. **b** Nodular aspect of the jejunal mucosa in a patient with pseudo-Whipple. **c** Pseudo-Whipple: Ziehl-Nielsen histologic examination, showing numerous acid-fast bacilli. **d.** Pseudo-Whipple: electron microscopy showing bacilli in lysosomial vesicles of macrophages

Chronic idiopathic ulcer of the small intestine in AIDS

First seen in the oropharynx, nonspecific ulcers in the esophagus were described later and, more recently, in the colon and small intestine. Among AIDS patients, cytomegalovirus and lymphoma are the most common etiologies, but tuberculosis, MAC, histoplasmosis, syphilis, Crohn's disease, adenocarcinoma and Kaposi's sarcoma have been reported. HIV itself seems to be the pathogenic agent.

Presentation is typically an intermittent small bowel obstruction in two-thirds of patients. Complications dominated by hemorrhage or perforation can reveal the disease in up to one-fourth of patients. Chronic anemia is also very common.

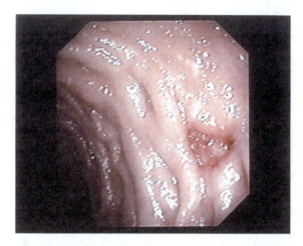

Fig. 5. Endoscopic aspect of chronic idiopathic ulcer of the small intestine in AIDS

Radiology

Barium examination may be useful, showing usually a unique ulcer (5 mm to - 3 cm in diameter), well delineated, with no surrounding edema, but a tendency to retraction and stenosis.

Endoscopy

Two-thirds of the ulcers are located in the distal ileum, but reports jejunal ulcers have been published recently. The lesion is deep, sometimes very large, with no surrounding inflammation and in some cases a visible vessel. Retraction of the bowel wall or stenosis is very common.

Histology

Pathologic examination of biopsies shows nonspecific ulceration surrounded by chronic and acute inflammatory cells. In some cases, HIV proteins or DNA have been found in the ulceration (Fig. 5).

Enteroscopy of the transplanted small bowel

C.L. Scotti-Foglieni, S.D. Tinozzi, K. Abu-Elmagd, T.E. Starzl

Introduction

The general term "intestinal/multivisceral transplantation" (InMvTx) refers to an heterogeneous class of transplants involving the whole small bowel (jejunum+ ileum), transplanted "en bloc" and simultaneously with or without one or more segments of the upper or lower gastrointestinal tract ("visceral component": stomach, duodenum, colon) and with or without one or more solid abdominal organs ("solid organ component": liver, pancreas, sometimes kidney/s).

The visceral and solid organ components of the intestinal/multivisceral graft may be transplanted in different combinations (Fig. 1), as required by the single recipient candidates:

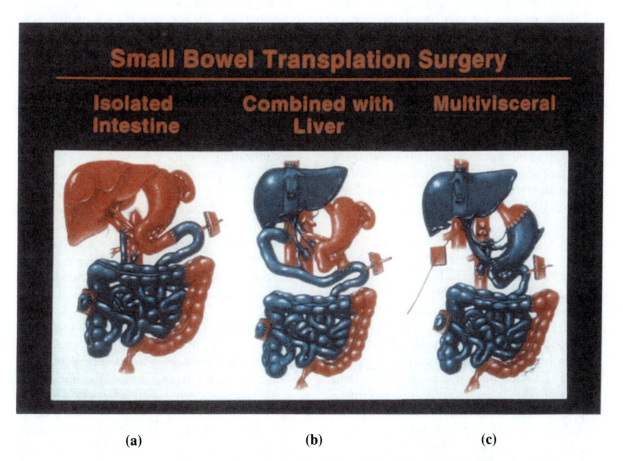

Fig. 1 a-c. The three different surgical types of intestinal and multivisceral transplanation: (**a**) isolated intestinal transplantation (iInTx); (**b**) combined liver and intestine transplantation (cLvInTx); (**c**) multivisceral transplantation (MvTx)

- Isolated intestine transplantation (iInTx):
  - Small bowel (SBTx)
  - Small bowel + colon (InTx)
- Combined liver and intestine tranplantation (cLvInTx):
  - Liver + small bowel (LvSBTx)
  - Liver + small bowel + colon (LvInTx)
- Multivisceral transplantation (MvTx):
  - Stomach + duodenum + liver + pancreas + intestine + (kidney/s)

Intestinal/multivisceral transplantation is usually indicated as a radical ultimate therapeutic option in the following two general clinical situations:

- for patients with chronic, irreversible end-stage intestinal failure, as an alternative and definitive treatment to unfeasible long-term TPN (relapsing TPN-induced complications: frequent line-related sepsis, extensive central vein thrombosis, exhaustion of the central venous access sites for TPN cannulation);
- for patients with otherwise normal intestine, but requiring simultaneous intestinal transplantation as an absolutely complementary surgical step, needed to replace different failed life-saving intra-abdominal solid organs (liver, pancreas).

More specifically, the indications for the different types of InMvTx (iInTx vs cLnInTx vs MvTx), as well as the various allograft organ configurations, rely on the anatomical integrity and on the functional status of the residual segments of the native gastrointestinal tract and of the native intra-abdominal solid organs (liver, pancreas). Such specific indications are summarized in Table 1.

Although attempted more than three decades ago, intestinal grafts have been considered until recently "forbidden organs" because of the high frequency of technical, immunological and infectious complications. It has been only since the advent of more refined harvesting and preservation procedures, of improved surgical techniques, of more effective immunosuppression (tacrolimus, mycophenolate/mofetil), and more sophisticated intra- and post-operative monitoring and treatment protocols that intestinal and multivisceral transplantation has become a clinical reality. However, the optimal management of InMvTx recipients still remains difficult and disputable, and major immunological or infectious complications still continue to pose threatening problems.

The post-operative course of InMvTx recipients is usually problematic and complicated, mainly in those patients who pre-operatively presented with severe deterioration of their physical performance status and with various organ system failures, which can persist and endure post-operatively even in the face of satisfactory allograft function. The post-operative course is usually more troubled in cLvInTx and in MvTx than in iInTx patients, who generally present a lesser medical acuity.

Consequently, post-operative monitoring and management of these patients require a very aggressive and multidisciplinary approach by the nursing and medical staff (surgeons, anesthesiologists, CCM physicians, internal medicine specialists, gastroenterologists and endoscopists, radiologists, pathologists).

It also requires easy availability and access to diagnostic facilities (immunologic and infectious surveillance, sophisticated hemodynamic monitoring, bronchoscopy, TEGraphy, non-invasive and invasive radiology, histopathology, emergency laboratory tests), as well as timely and prompt therapeutic modalities (immunosuppressive and immunodulation management, antibiotic therapy, mechanical ventilation and respiratory treatment, hemodialysis, fluid and nutritional support, emergency surgery for complications, etc.).

Most important, however, is a continuous, dedicated, diligent commitment to patient surveillance and care by medical, surgical and nursing personnel: any subjective symptom or complaint, as well as any new objective physical sign or change in the patient's clinical picture (Table 2 A, B), must be aggressively pursued and carefully investigated until the cause is found or it resolves.

Although sometimes difficult to achieve, early diagnosis of post-operative complications is a major determinant in successful InMvTx, being a "conditio sine qua non" for immediate, specific, effective therapy. Post-operative monitoring of InMvTx recipients is addressed to detect as early as possible the onset of post-transplant complications, mainly immunological and infectious, as well as to assess the intestinal graft's anatomic and functional integrity

Table 1. Indications for intestinal/multivisceral transplantation

TRANSPLANTATION TYPE	INDICATIONS

ISOLATED INTESTINAL TRANSPLANTATION (iInTx)	1) SURGICAL "SHORT GUT SYNDROME" (loss ≥ 80%):
	  a) in adult patients:
	    • abdominal trauma
	    • vascular diseases involving the CA[1] and/or the SMA[2]
	    • multiple extensive intestinal resections for surgical adhesions from previous surgeries
	    • Crohn's disease
	    • Gardner's syndrome
	    • incarcerating intra-abdominal desmoid tumors
	  b) in pediatric patients:
	    • intestinal atresia
	    • gastroschisis
	    • mid-gut volvulus
	    • necrotizing enterocolitis
	2) CHRONIC PSEUDO-OBSTRUCTION SYNDROMES: from
	    • visceral myopathy
	    • visceral neuropathy
	    • total intestinal agangliosis
	3) SEVERE ENTEROCYTE ABSORTIVE/SECRETORY DYSFUNCTION: from
	    • microvillous inclusion disease
	    • radiation enteritis
	    • diffuse inflammatory bowel disease
	    • massive intestinal polyposis syndromes
	    • protein-losing enteropathy

COMBINED HEPATIC/INTESTINAL TRANSPLANTATION (cLvInTx)	1) COEXISTENT INTESTINAL & HEPATIC FAILURE: from
	    • short gut syndrome +
	    • long-term TPN[3]-induced end-stage liver disease
	2) OLTx[4] CANDIDATES WITH CONCOMITANT EXTENSIVE THROMBOSIS OF THE ENTIRE PORTOMESENTERIC VENOUS SYSTEM (requiring total enterectomy of otherwise normally functioning intestine)

MULTIVISCERAL TRANSPLANTATION (MvTx)	1) COEXISTENT TERMINAL INTESTINAL, HEPATIC, PANCREATIC DISEASE: from extensive thrombosis of the splanchnic and/or inferior vena cava systems, due to
	    • congenital protein C deficiency
	    • congenital protein S deficiency
	    • congenital anti-thrombin III deficiency
	2) LOW-MALIGNANT DIFFUSE INTRA-ABDOMINAL TUMORS:
	    • diffuse polyposis syndromes
	    • desmoid tumors
	3) POTENTIALLY CURABLE MALIGNANCIES: requiring upper abdominal exenteration
	    • gastrinoma
	    • carcinoid
	4) SEVERE GI MOTILITY DISORDERS:
	    • myogenic pseudo-obstruction syndrome
	    • neurogenic pseudo-obstruction syndrome

[1]CA: celiac axis; [2]SMA: superior mesenteric artery; [3]TPN: total parenteral nutrition; [4]OLTx: orthotopic liver transplantation

Table 2. Pre-endoscopic and endoscopic findings in intestinal/multivisceral transplantation

A. PRE-ENDOSCOPIC SYMPTOMS	B. PRE-ENDOSCOPIC PHYSICAL SIGNS	C. ENDOSCOPIC FINDINGS & DESCRIPTIVE ENDOSCOPIC VOCABULARY

• fever
• chills
• weight loss
• mood changes
• abdominal distension
• abdominal pain
• anorexia
• dysphagia
• odynophagia
• regurgitation
• heartburn
• nausea
• vomiting
• constipation
• diarrhea
• intestinal bleeding
• melena
• hematochezia
	• fever
	• sepsis, septic shock
	• ARDS-like syndrome
	• toxemia
	• malnutrition
	• dehydration
	• weight loss
	• abdominal distension
	• abdominal tenderness
	• abdominal muscular spasticity/rigidity
	• stomal appearance
	• high stomal output
	• diarrhea
	• intestinal bleeding
	  – occult
	  – melena
	  – hematochezia
	• alterations in bowel movement habits:
	  – obstipation/constipation
	  – obstruction
	  – paralytic ileus
		• mucosal findings & distribution (punctate, spotty, patchy, segmental, diffuse):
		  – velvety, glistening appearance
		  – erythema
		  – hyperemia
		  – apparent vascularity
		  – edema
		  – pale, ischemic appearance
		  – congested, dusky, cyanotic appearance
		  – granularity
		  – nodularity
		  – friability
		  – sloughing of the mucosa
		  – erosion
		  – ulcer
		  – exudate
		  – pseudomembrane
		  – thickening of the mucosa
		  – flattening or atrophy of the mucosal folds
		  – stiffness and tubular appearance of the loop
		• luminal content:
		  – feces consistency and appearance
		  – stomal output
		    – increased
		    – decreased
		  – loose stools
		  – watery diarrhea
		  – intestinal bleeding, melena, hematochezia
		• intestinal loop motility:
		  – hypoperistalsis, hypokinesis
		  – paralytic ileus
		  – hyperperistalsis

(absorption, motility, fluid and electrolyte balance, nutritional status).

Unlike heart, kidney, pancreas and liver transplantation, the intestine (as well as the lung), is the only organ which can be endoscopically explored and monitored after transplantation for major immunological (acute cellular rejection, chronic rejection, graft-versus-host disease) or infectious complications (CMV enteritis, EBV infection with PTLD, mycotic enteritis). While the diagnosis of infection is relatively easy and clear-cut, monitoring of the intestinal graft for immunological complications (mainly acute cellular rejection) is difficult and disputable because there are no clearly defined specific clinical and laboratory parameters known to be reliable and of value. Consequently, enteroscopy, endoscopy-guided biopsies, endoscopic medication and surgery of the graft can play a critical role and be, together with histopathology, the cornerstone of post-operative monitoring and management of intestinal/multivisceral transplant recipients.

Enteroscopy methodologies and procedures in intestinal/multivisceral transplantation recipients

Indications for intestinal graft enteroscopy

The indications for enteroscopic evaluation include routine surveillance (25%) or the onset of pre-endoscopic clinical symptoms (Table 2 A) or pre-endoscopic physical signs (Table 2 B) (75%), consistent with the initial outbreak of major complications.

More accurately, the most frequent clinical indications for intestinal graft endoscopy in adult InMvTx recipients are: abdominal pain (72%), increased stomal output (46%), abdominal distension (30%), nausea (20%), fever (17%), vomiting (10%), intestinal bleeding (10%) and sepsis (4%).

In pediatric InMvTx patients, the most frequent indications for the enteroscopies are: fever, change in stomal output and appearance, gastro-intestinal bleeding and others (sepsis, skin rash, etc.).

Enteroscopic procedures

The enteroscopic procedures performed in recipients of intestinal/multivisceral transplants differ in some aspects from the standard methodologies and protocols utilized in non-transplanted patients.

Because of the frequent patchy or segmental topographic anatomic distribution of the immunological and/or infectious lesions in the mucosa of the different intestinal segments of the transplanted graft (stomach, duodenum, jejunum, ileum, colon), the enteroscopic procedure should explore as much gastrointestinal tract as possible in order to avoid "skip" lesions and minimize underevaluation of the initial and ongoing complications.

Enteroscopies are usually performed mainly by trans-stomal terminal ileoscopy or trans-stomal ileocolonoscopy(63%), but also by trans-stomal jejunoscopy (4%), esophagogastroduodenoscopy (23%), and lower proctosigmoid colonoscopy (10%).

Routine surveillance enteroscopies are done twice a week for the 1st month, once a week for the next 2 months, monthly for the next 3 months and every 3-6 months thereafter.

In addition, whenever the evolving clinical picture of the InMvTx recipients (Table 2 A, B) is consistent with the onset of major complications, timely turning to gastroenteroscopy is absolutely mandatory.

Because data which define the endoscopic appearance of the intestinal graft or that correlate the symptoms and signs of rejection and/or infection with concurrent graft endoscopic appearance are still lacking or inadequately outlined, a standardized enteroscopic descriptive vocabulary referring to endoscopic features found in transplanted intestinal grafts complicated by immunological or infectious events has been developed and presented herein (Table 2 C). The aim of this standardized enteroscopic descriptive vocabulary is to accomplish easily identifiable features and terms with a high degree of reproducibility, as well as to minimize the examiner variations, thus increasing the value and reliability of the overall endoscopic examination as a diagnostic tool for intestinal and multivisceral graft complications.

The endoscopic procedures performed in patients with intestinal and multivisceral transplantation should be frequently captured and saved on videotape to generate an enteroscopic video-library, thus allowing the comparative assessment of previous and subsequent enteroscopic features, as well as the endoscopic evaluation of the clinical course of the intestinal/multivisceral transplant.

Since the histopathologic diagnosis is still considered the gold standard for comparison, enteroscopic evaluation should not be used as the sole and exclusive tool in diagnosing immunological and infectious complications; consequently, enteroscopy must be routinely associated with multiple, selective, endoscopy-guided mucosal biopsies.

Monitoring of immunological and infectious complications in human clinical intestinal and multivisceral transplantation

In monitoring post-operative immunological and infectious complications in intestinal and multivisceral transplantation recipients, the indication to enteroscopic evaluation is based mainly on clinical criteria (Table 2 A, B). Furthermore, the sensitivity, specificity, positive or negative predictive value and diagnostic accuracy of using the endoscopic findings (Table 2 C) as predictors of the immunological or infectious complications in the intestinal/multivisceral graft have yet to be fully established. As a matter of fact, complete endoscopic surveillance of all gastroenteric segments of the transplanted graft for diagnostic purpose or for biopsy sampling is not always feasible or safe. Additionally, in the intestinal graft acute cellular rejection lesions are unevenly distributed in a spotty or segmental fashion, often ileal-centered, thus making endoscopy problematic and unsafe to be performed. Moreover, several frequent endoscopic findings (edema, erythema, erosions, ulcers) are not specific, being found both in immunological (ACR) and in infectious (CMV enteritis) complications. Consequently, because of these methodological limitations, enteroscopy should not be the sole unique diagnostic tool, but it has to be always compared with an available reference gold standard, ideally represented by the histopathologic examination. In the clinical setting, histopathology may be not always available, so the following alternative diagnostic options should be used, such as comparison and correlation of enteroscopic and histopathological findings with clinical assessment and outcome, as well as with imaging criteria.

Clinical findings

Clinical monitoring of the intestinal graft is accomplished by multiple daily clinical evaluations, focusing on the patient's general clinical status and on the patterns of the intestinal stoma (Table 2 A,B).

Acute intestinal allograft rejection

Acute intestinal allograft rejection (Fig. 2) may be asymptomatic, but usually presents an array of symptoms and physical signs (Table 2 A, B), including fever, weakness, mood changes, abdominal pain, abdominal distension, hypoperistalsis and paralytic ileus, nausea and vomiting, diarrhea or sudden increase of watery stomal discharge.

The intestinal graft stoma (usually an ileostomy) is carefully examined for color, texture and friability of the mucosa; the stoma may progressively become edematous, erythematous, pale, congested, dusky and friable.

Stomal output is assessed for volume, consistency, presence of blood and of reducing substances, tested by pH and clinitest, and reflecting, besides rejection, also infection and malab-

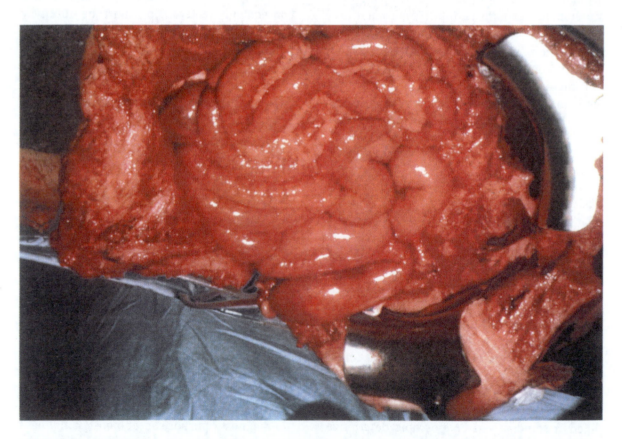

Fig. 2. Gross appearance of early acute cellular rejection in an isolated small bowel allograft: the recipient has been surgically explored because of fever, sepsis, ARDS-like syndrome, abdominal pain, abdominal distension, hypoperistalsis and increase of watery stomal discharge. The intestinal loops look erythematous, edematous, slightly distended, hypokynetic

sorption. In more severe episodes of acute graft rejection, erosions, ulcerations and sloughing of the intestinal mucosa may occur, with gastrointestinal bleeding, graft paralytic ileus and decrease or absence of stomal discharge.

Due to disruption of the normal intestinal mucosal barrier, bacterial and/or fungal translocation can develop, with consequent sepsis, septic shock and/or ARDS-like syndromes.

Clinical criteria are the keystone for early diagnosis of acute rejection of the intestinal graft. Unlike rejection of other isolated solid organ allografts (heart, lung, liver, kidney, pancreas), whose diagnosis is mainly attained by biopsy and/or by functional or laboratory tests, diagnosis of intestinal acute rejection has to be primarily based on clinical criteria, which usually present first. In InMvTx endoscopic, bioptic, radiological and metabolic parameters of acute rejection often come too late: they help to confirm, not to make the primary diagnosis of acute rejection. It would be an unforgivable mistake and a waste of precious time if we were to wait too long for these results to start immunosuppressive treatment, since only a few hours may be available for effectively and safely reversing the ongoing immunological injury.

Chronic intestinal allograft rejection

Chronic rejection of intestinal allografts (Fig. 3) has been recorded in recipients with persistent or recurrent intractable acute rejection episodes. Clinical presentation consists of chronic progressive allograft dysfunction with intermittent fever, worsening malnutrition, weight loss, chronic long-lasting exacerbating abdominal pain, recurrent or persistent intractable diarrhea with dehydration, intermittent melena or enterorrhagia, relapsing septic episodes.

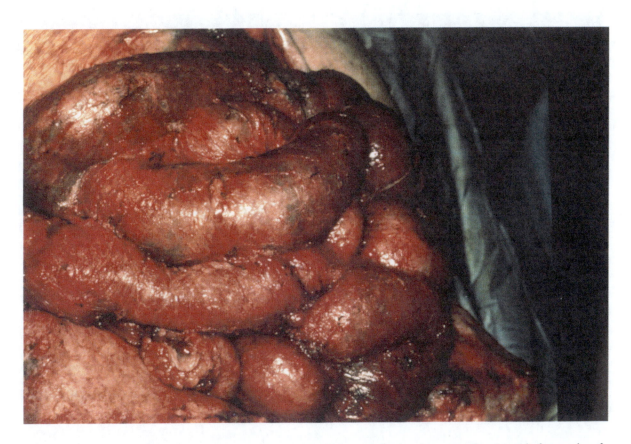

Fig. 3. Macroscopic aspect of an isolated intestinal allograft with chronic rejection: intraoperative picture before total graft enterectomy and retransplantation after 667 days since the primary iInTx. The recipient's clinical course consisted of reccurrent acute rejection episodes, with progressive allograft dysfunction, relapsing septic episodes, intermittent fever, malnutrition, weight loss, exacerbating abdominal pain, refractory diarrhea with dehydration, melena. The intestinal loops show a rigid, stiff, tubular, hypokinetic appearance, with segmental strictures and dilations, along with ischemic areas and intestinal perforations

Graft-versus-host disease

The clinical picture of the infrequently occurring graft-versus-host disease episodes (5%) include fever, skin rash, septic-like syndrome, abdominal pain and distension, changes in the stomal appearance and output.

Infectious complications

Clinical presentation of infectious complications varies with the infectious etiologic pathogens. Bacterial infections clinically present mostly as line sepsis, pneumonia, wound and intra-abdominal abscesses.

Fungal infections occur in the esophagus, peritoneal cavity, paranasal sinuses, upper and lower respiratory system.

Viral infections present in adults mainly as CMV enteritis; other clinical pictures consist of CMV hepatitis, pneumonitis, gastritis, retinitis and diffuse CMV syndrome. Pediatric recipients seem more prone to EBV infections (PTLD and acute lymphadenitis), which should be suspected when clinical symptoms and signs including fever, abdominal pain, bleeding and/or vomiting occur. These features vary according to the location of the lesions, their size and the depth of mucosal invasion. PTLD can be further complicated by acute cellular rejection, owing to reduced immunosuppression required to treat the lymphoproliferative disease. Moreover, PTLD may be complicated by sepsis and toxemia, secondary to the entrance of the enteric flora and toxins through the disrupted mucosal barrier.

Exclusive infectious clinical and physiopathological features occurring in this unique

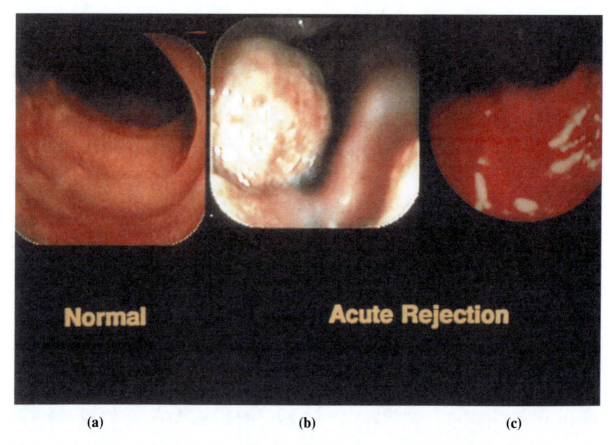

Fig. 4 a-c. Enteroscopic appearance of an isolated intestinal allograft with acute cellular rejection: (a) reference picture of a normal intestinal allograft (ileum); (b) early moderate acute cellular rejection: the mucosa is edematous, has lost its peculiar glistening and velvety appearance, is friable, with submucosal nodularity and small mucosal ulcers; (c) severe acute cellular rejection: the intestinal mucosa shows diffuse erosions with sloughing of extensive areas of its superficial layer, intestinal bleeding and paralytic ileus (by courtesy of Lippincot-Raven Publishers, Philadelphia, USA; from: Fung JJ, Abu-Elmagd K and Todo S: Intestinal and Multivisceral Transplantation. In: *Digestive Tract Surgery: a Text and Atlas*, Fig. 35.15, p. 1242)

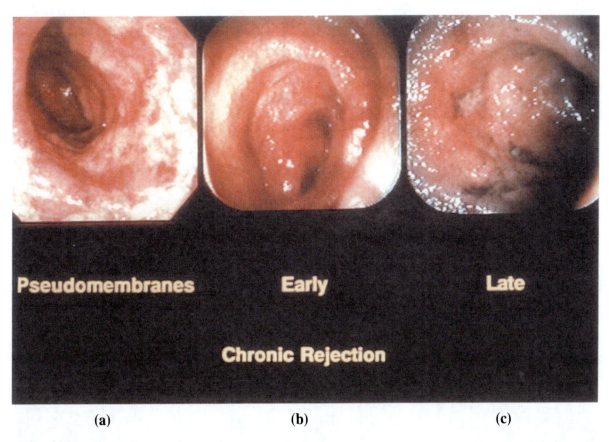

Fig. 5 a-c. Enteroscopic appearance of an isolated intestinal allograft with chronic rejection: (a) early chronic intestinal allograft rejection: the mucosa shows submucosal nodularity, focal erosions with development of pseudomembranes; (b) early chronic intestinal allograft rejection: hypokinetic appearance of the intestinal loop, with edema of the mucosa, flattening of the mucosal folds, fine mucosal granularity with submucosal nodularity and focal erosions; (c) late phase of severe chronic intestinal allograft rejection: rigid, tubular, akinetic appearance of the intestinal loop, with thickening of the mucosa, atrophy of the mucosal folds, chronic ulcerations with intestinal bleeding (by courtesy of Lippincot-Raven Publishers, Philadelphia, USA; from: Fung JJ, Abu-Elmagd K and Todo S: Intestinal and Multivisceral Transplantation. In: *Digestive Tract Surgery: a Text and Atlas*, Fig. 35.117, p. 1243)

patient population are microbial overgrowth and translocation.

In addition to daily infectious surveillance tests routinely performed in any transplant patient, infection monitoring of InMvTx recipients should include frequent cultures of the blood, sputum, bronchial and alveolar secretions, urine, surgical wound exudate and drains' fluid. Most important are quantitative cultures of the stools and of the stomal discharge in order to monitor significant changes in the intestinal microflora and to confirm direct correlation between the onset of systemic infectious episodes and the simultaneously ongoing microbial overgrowth and translocation processes.

In all cases of sepsis of unexplained origin in any InMvTx recipient, the basic general principle of endoscopically and radiologically exploring each of the surgical anastomoses (gastrointestinal, biliary, vascular) by different enteroscopic procedures and by ultrasound, Doppler sonography, CT scan, angiography, barium contrast series, PTC, etc. is paramount and should always be promptly considered and timely performed.

Endoscopic findings

Acute intestinal allograft rejection

Endoscopic features of mild-to-moderate acute intestinal graft rejection are edema of the mucosa, which can progressively become focally or diffusely erythematous, hyperemic, congested and dusky. It can lose its fine, glistening and velvety appearance and become hypoperistaltic, friable, with fine mucosal granularity and focal erosions (Fig. 4b). More severe rejection presents with submucosal nodularity, focal or diffuse ulcerations, sloughing of extensive areas of the mucosa with development of pseudomembranes, intestinal bleeding and absence of peristalsis (Fig. 4c).

Chronic intestinal allograft rejection

Chronic intestinal allograft rejection in its early course can show features similar to those enteroscopically found in late ongoing or relapsing acute cellular rejection of the intestinal allograft (Fig. 5b).

Endoscopic examination of late chronic intestinal allograft rejection shows a rigid, stiff, tubular, hypokinetic appearance of the intestinal loops, with thickening of the mucosa, flattening or atrophy of the mucosal folds, chronic ulcerations with pseudomembranes and intestinal bleeding (Fig. 5c).

Infectious complications

Differential endoscopic diagnosis should be made between acute cellular rejection of the intestinal graft and CMV enteritis occurring mostly in adult recipients, and intestinal PTLD presenting mainly in pediatric patients.

The endoscopic features of CMV enteritis include punctuate areas of erythema, spotty mucosal erosions and focal ulcerations (Fig. 6a).

Fungal enteritis endoscopically shows superficial, white, curdy patches, sometimes growing together into large, soft and light membranes. These are easily removed, leaving an erythema-

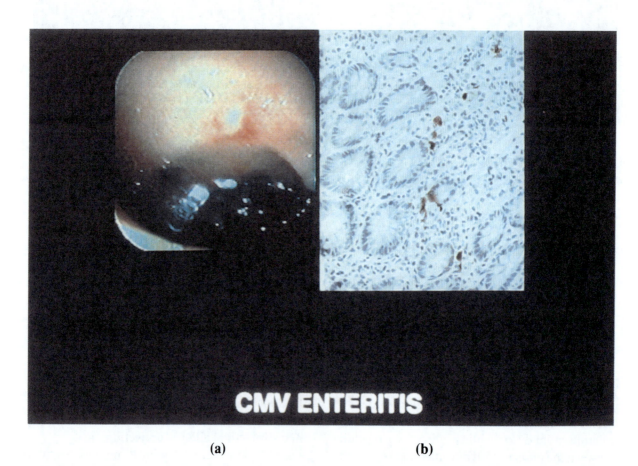

(a) (b)

Fig. 6 a,b. Cytomegalovirus enteritis in an intestinal allograft: (a) endoscopic picture: the mucosa shows edema, punctate areas of erythema and focal mucosal erosion; (b) histopathologic picture: giant mucosal epithelial cells, with pleomorphic nuclei, basophilic nuclear and cytoplasmic inclusion bodies, mixed inflammatory cell infiltrate, cryptitis

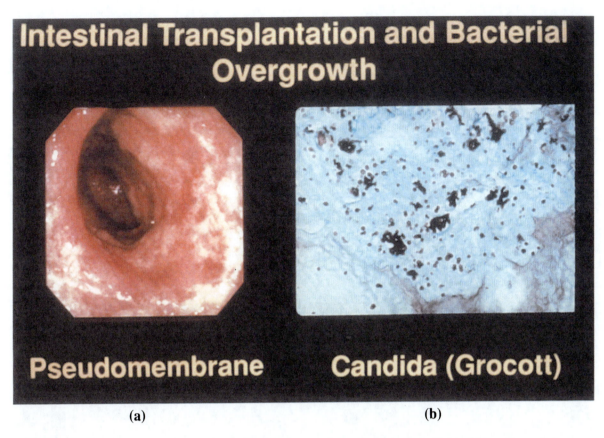

Fig. 7 a,b. *Candida albicans* enteritis in an intestinal allograft: (a) endoscopic picture: superficial, white, curdy patches growing into light pseudomembranes, with erythematous, inflamed surrounding and underlying mucosa; (b) histopathologic picture: yeasts and pseudohyphae within the pseudomembrane and the underlying mucosal epithelial layer

Table 3. Histopathological findings in InMvTx immunological complications

ACUTE CELLULAR REJECTION	CHRONIC REJECTION
a) early, mild to moderate ACR: • widening of the lamina propria • edema • mixed inflammatory mononuclear infiltrate (large activated lymphoblasts, small lymphocytes, macrophages, plasma cells, eosinophils, neutrophil granulocytes, • focal endothelialitis • infiltration of the basal membrane and of the epithelium • cryptitis with apoptosis • goblet and Paneth cell depletion • epithelial cell necrosis • crypt loss b) late, advanced, severe ACR: • mucosal sloughing • focal ulcerations • crypt destruction • neutrophil plugging of capillaries • granulation tissue • inflammatory pseudomembranes c) healing and regeneration changes: • architecture disruption • doubling of the epithelial monolayer • distorted, uneven cryptic lumen • villous blunting	a) early, moderate chronic rejection: • progressive distortion of the mucosal architecture • villous blunting • widening of the lamina propria • scant cellular infiltrate • severe prominent cryptitis • cryptic cell apoptosis • depletion or loss of goblet and Paneth cells b) advanced, severe chronic rejection: • focal chronic ulcerations • mucosal microabscesses • epithelial metaplasia • fibrosis of the lamina propria • fibrosis of the submucosa • fibrosis of the mesenteric lymph nodes • obliterative arteriopathy of the intestinal arterioles

tous, irritated, inflamed underlying mucosal surface (Fig. 7a).

Endoscopically, PTLD early lesions are not specific, consisting of non-ulcerated nodules of the submucosa, covered by the overlying mucosal layer with or without concurrent erythema. In contrast, well-developed PTLD lesions are peculiar, represented by submucosal nodules up to 2 cm in diameter, with deep necrotic central areas surrounded by heaped-up mucosa.

Histopathological findings

Histopathological criteria (Table 3) are the gold standard reference, with which clinical, enteroscopic and radiological findings should be compared. Specific histological criteria for acute cellular rejection (mild, moderate, severe), chronic rejection (early, late), based on extension of inflammatory infiltrate, severity of crypt cell damage and apoptosis, focal or diffuse ulceration, severity of intestinal mucosal architecture

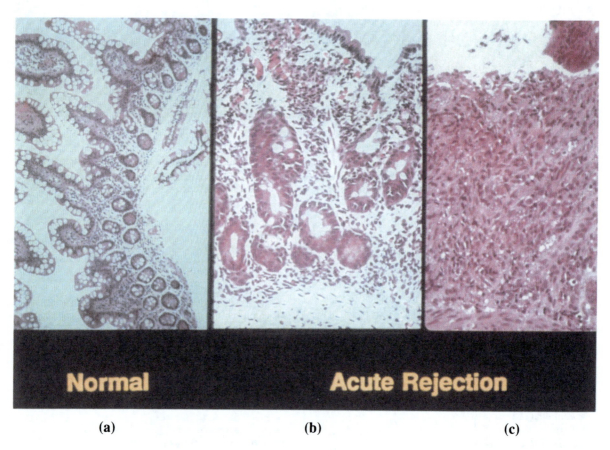

(a) (b) (c)

Fig. 8 a-c. Histopathology of intestinal allograft acute cellular rejection: (a) reference picture of a normal intestinal allograft; (b) early mild acute cellular rejection: the major histopathological patterns include widening of the lamina propria, with edema, mononuclear cellular infiltrate, capillary congestion with endothelialitis, significant crypt damage (cryptitis) with infiltration of the basal membrane and of the mucosal epithelial layer, depletion of goblet and Paneth cells, epithelial cell necrosis; (c) advanced and severe uncontrolled acute cellular rejection: the endoscopy-guided superficial biopsy shows a thick, mixed pleomorphic inflammatory infiltrate of the lamina propria and submucosa, massive crypt loss, blunting of the villi, mucosal sloughing with pseudomembranes and widespread mucosal destruction. The cellular infiltrate components are mainly large activated lymphoblasts and small lymphocytes, along with macrophages, plasmacells, eosinophils and sometimes neutrophil granulocytes (by courtesy of Lippincot-Raven Publishers, Philadelphia, USA; from: Fung JJ, Abu-Elmagd K and Todo S: Intestinal and Multivisceral Transplantation. In: *Digestive Tract Surgery: a Text and Atlas*, Fig. 35.116, p. 1243)

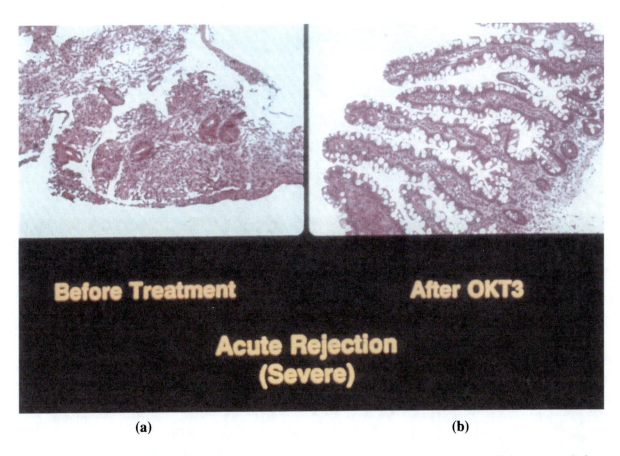

Fig. 9 a,b. Histopathology of intestinal allograft acute cellular rejection: (a) ongoing severe acute cellular rejection before treatment: the histological picture includes mixed pleomorphic inflammatory infiltrate of the lamina propria, cryptitis and crypt loss, complete mucosal sloughing with focal ulceration and replacing granulation tissue and pseudomembranes, disruption of the normal enteric mucosal architecture; (b) after timely, aggressive and successful treatment of the ongoing acute cellular rejection episode, owing to the peculiar regenerative capacities of the enteric mucosa, it can revert to an almost normal histological structure. Histological healing comes late, usually 5-7 days after the clinically improving response

distortion, as well as for graft-versus-host disease and infectious lesions (namely, CMV and EBV injuries) in the transplanted intestinal allograft, are now available with adequate accuracy.

Acute intestinal allograft rejection

In mild to moderate rejection (Fig. 8), histopathological criteria consist of widening of the lamina propria, with edema, mixed inflammatory mononuclear infiltrate and focal endothelialitis (inflammatory cells adherent to or infiltrating the injured endothelium).

The cellular infiltrate components are mainly activated lymphoblasts and small lymphocytes, along with macrophages, plasma cells, eosinophils and sometimes neutrophil granulocytes.

The cellular infiltrate can traverse the muscularis mucosae as well as invade the basal membrane, with resultant infiltration of the mucosal epithelial layer.

Cryptitis with apoptosis, goblet and Paneth cell depletion, epithelial cell necrosis and final crypt loss of various degrees are further histologic findings of mild to moderate acute intestinal rejection.

At a more advanced and severe stage (Fig. 9), complete mucosal sloughing, focal ulcerations, crypt destruction, neutrophil plugging of capillaries, replacing granulation tissue and inflammatory pseudomembranes are found.

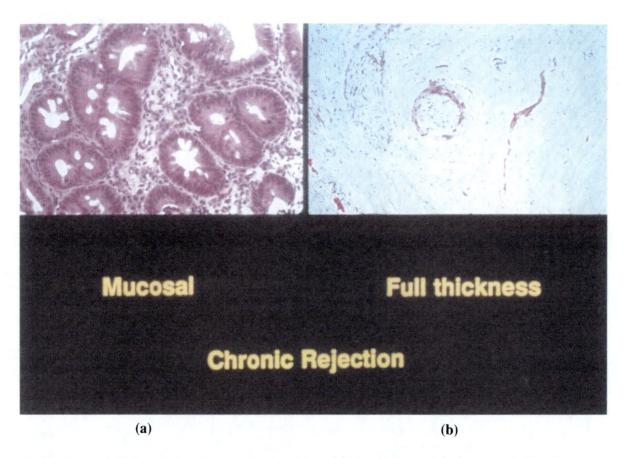

Fig. 10 a,b. Histopathology of intestinal allograft chronic rejection: (a) endoscopic-guided superficial mucosal biopsy includes progressive distortion of the mucosal architecture, villous blunting, widening and fibrosis of the lamina propria with scan cellular infiltrate, prominent cryptitis with crypt loss; (b) full-thickness intestinal biopsy shows chronic obliterative arteriopathy of the intestinal arterioles

Healing and regeneration changes occur, overlapping the above histopathologic features, with resulting architecture disruption, doubling of the epithelial monolayer, distorted, uneven cryptic lumen and villous blunting.

It should be stressed that histopathologic features of intestinal acute rejection can be focal or segmental, often localized in the ileum.

Histologic differential diagnosis is often difficult and should be formulated for intestinal graft ischemic injury and CMV enteritis. Ischemic (harvesting, preservation and reperfusion) injury of the intestinal graft usually occurs after 7.5 h of cold ischemia time and consists of focal epithelial denudation of the villi along with congestion or hemorrhage in the lamina propria. These lesions, when reversible, usually heal within 10 days after transplantation.

Chronic intestinal allograft rejection

Histologically, on endoscopic-guided mucosal biopsies, there is a progressive distortion of the mucosal architecture, with villous blunting, widening of the lamina propria, scant cellular infiltrate, severe prominent cryptitis with cryptic cell apoptosis, depletion or loss of goblet and Paneth cells.

In more severe and advanced stages, focal chronic ulcerations, mucosal microabscesses, epithelial metaplasia, fibrosis of the lamina propria, of the submucosa and of the mesenteric lymph nodes (Fig. 10a), along with obliterative arteriopathy of the intestinal arterioles occur, as demonstrated by full-thickness intestinal biopsies (Fig. 10b).

Graft-versus-host disease
Pathologic monitoring of GVHD is by standard histology, immunohistochemical techniques [immunostaining, sex identification after fluorescence-in-situ hybridization (FISH) and PCR karyotyping ("DNA fingerprinting")]. With these procedures it is possible to differentiate migrating immunocompetent cells of the donor (donor "passenger leukocytes") from recipient cells, as well as to document the immunological injury of the recipient tissue by the donor-infiltrating cells. Inadequate immunosuppression is a major risk factor for GVHD. In spite of the historical fear of a high incidence of GVHD, documented in experimental intestinal transplantation, recent clinical experience has actually shown minor GVHD occurrence (5%).

One of the most intriguing findings from the above analyses is the gradual replacement of the donor hematolymphoid cells in the intestinal wall and mesenteric lymph nodes of the graft by immunocompetent hematolymphoid cells from the recipient (recipient "passenger leukocytes"), which rearrange the normal intestinal mucosal immune system architecture. Conversely, donor migratory immunocytes (donor "passenger leukocytes") from the graft migrate at the same time ubiquitously into the recipient's blood stream and tissues. This new immunological status ("systemic microchimerism") could be the basis of gradual induction of future donor-specific non-reactivity ("tolerance").

Infectious enteritis
Major histologic features of CMV enteritis are giant mucosal epithelial cells with pleomorphic nuclei, harboring basophilic nuclear and cytoplasmic inclusion bodies, mixed inflammatory cell infiltrate, cryptitis, epithelial cell necrosis, apoptosis and villous atrophy (Fig. 6b).

In invasive *Candida* enteritis, subsequent to disruption of the mucosal barrier, histopathological findings show the yeasts or pseudohyphal forms of the fungus within the epithelial layer, the lamina propria or the submucosa (Fig. 7b). Sometimes, in severe and advanced cases, invasive enteric candidiasis is characterized by the presence of microabscesses, with the yeast at the center of the lesion, with a surrounding area of inflammatory cell infiltrate and necrosis.

Imaging findings

Acute intestinal allograft rejection
Radiological criteria are based on gastrointestinal contrast studies, CT scan and gastrointestinal transit and emptying-time evaluations. They consist of enlargement of the intestinal lumen, edema and thickening of the intestinal wall, blunting and loss of the mucosal folds, and paralytic ileus with increased transit and emptying times (Fig. 11).

Chronic intestinal allograft rejection
Radiologically, intestinal contrast studies show a stiff, rigid, tubular appearance of the intestinal loops, sometimes with strictures, flattening or loss of the mucosal folds, paralytic ileus with resultant increased transit and emptying times (Fig. 12a).

CT scans exhibit the same picture as above, with significant thickening of the intestinal mucosa.

Angiography has revealed segmental stenosis of the mesenteric arterioles (Fig. 12b), validating the obliterative arteriopathy of the delayed long-lasting chronic rejecting intestinal graft (Fig. 10b).

Conclusions

Although human clinical intestinal and multivisceral transplantation has recently become a feasible treatment for patients with chronic, irreversible, end-stage intestinal failure (Table 1), monitoring and management of their early and late post-operative course still remain problematic due to the frequent onset of severe early and late immunological and infectious complications.

Monitoring of the intestinal graft for rejection (mainly ACR) is often difficult and questionable because there are no clearly defined specific clinical and laboratory parameters known to be reliable and of value. Consequently, enteroscopy, endoscopy-guided biopsies,

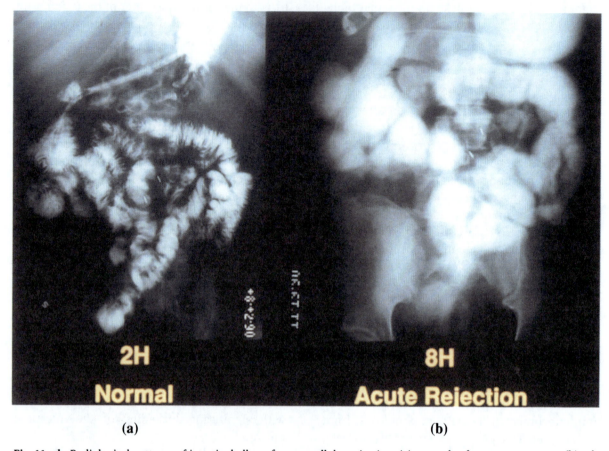

Fig. 11 a,b. Radiological patterns of intestinal allograft acute cellular rejection: (a) normal reference appearance; (b) 8 h after the onset of the first clinical symptoms and signs, contrast studies of the transplanted isolated intestinal allograft show dilation of the intestinal lumen, edema and thickening of the intestinal wall, blunting and loss of the mucosal folds, and paralytic ileus with increased transit and emptying times

endoscopic medication and surgery of the graft can play a critical role.

Since the gastrointestinal tract, as well as the lungs, are the only organs which can be visually explored following transplantation, post-transplant monitoring and treatment could be facilitated by looking directly at the gastrointestinal mucosal appearance endoscopically, as well as by obtaining enteroscopically guided mucosal biopsies for histopathology and cultures.

Conversely, enteroscopy of the transplanted intestinal/multivisceral graft still presents some methodological limitations: total endoscopic surveillance of all gastroenteric segments of the entire transplanted graft for diagnostic purposes or for biopsy sampling is not always feasible or safe.

In the intestinal graft, acute cellular rejection lesions are unevenly distributed in a spotty or segmental fashion, often ileal-centered, thus making endoscopy problematic and unsafe to be performed.

Little data exist that define with an appropriate descriptive vocabulary the endoscopic appearance of the intestinal graft and that correlate the properly characterized endoscopic picture of the graft with symptoms and signs of rejection or infection, as well as with the temporal sequence of treatment and clinical evolution of InMvTx recipients. Acceptable reproducibility of the overall endoscopic examination is required to minimize the level of examiner variability and to raise the diagnostic yield of the enteroscopic procedures.

Several frequently encountered endoscopic findings (edema, erythema, erosions, ulcers) are

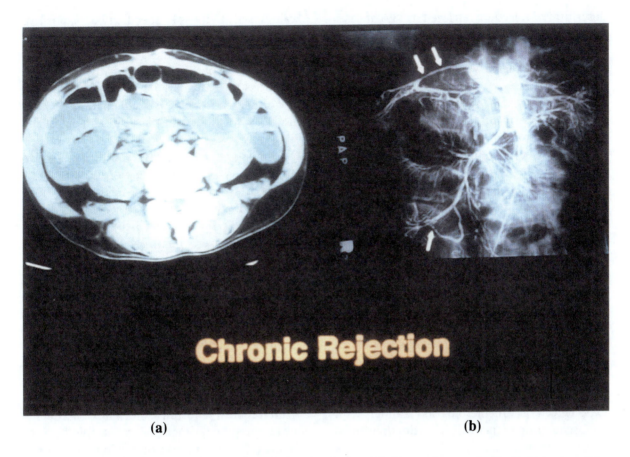

Fig. 12 a,b. "Imaging" features of intestinal allograft chronic rejection: (a) CT scan shows a significant thickening of the intestinal mucosa and of the entire intestinal wall, a stiff, rigid, tubular appearance of the intestinal loops, sometimes with strictures, flattening or loss of the mucosal folds, paralytic ileus with increased transit and emptying times; (b) superior mesentric artery angiography discloses segmental stenosis of the marginal mesenteric arterioles (*arrows*), validating the obliterative arteriopathy of the late chronic rejecting intestinal graft (by courtesy of Lippincot-Raven Publishers, Philadelphia, USA; from: Fung JJ, Abu-Elmagd K and Todo S: Intestinal and Multivisceral Transplantation. In: *Digestive Tract Surgery: a Text and Atlas*, Fig. 35.19, 35.20, p. 1244)

not specific, as both are found in immunological (ACR) and infectious (CMV enteritis) complications.

Finally, the sensitivity, specificity, positive or negative predictive value and diagnostic accuracy of using the endoscopic findings as predictors of the immunological or infectious complications in the intestinal/multivisceral graft have yet to be fully established.

Actually, the endoscopic gross appearance does not always correlate with the endoscopy-guided histopathological findings: Garau et al. have demonstrated that rejection was histologically confirmed in 4 of 91 (4%) procedures with endoscopically normal mucosa, in 6 (9%) of 64 procedures with endoscopic features of inflammation (hyperemia, edema friability, loss of mucosal folds), and in 4 of 29 (14%) of those with endoscopic findings of ulceration.

Hassanein et al. have shown that the only symptom and sign that significantly ($p < 0.05$) correlated with rejection was fever. Similarly, high stomal discharge was very consistent with rejection and very seldom was secondary to CMV infection. On enteroscopic examination, a glistening or velvety appearance of the mucosa, the presence of normal mucosal folds and of normal mucosal vascular patterns were strongly suggestive of a healthy graft. Conversely, mucosal erythema, erosions, ulcers and pseudomembranes were never considered normal: mucosal erythema was a significant descriptor of rejection, retrieved in 78% of cases of ACR; diffuse ulceration was found in 33% of cases of rejection; focal ulceration with punctuate areas of erythema was a critical sign of CMV enteritis.

Enteroscopy and endoscopy-guided biopsies are valuable in monitoring InMvTx recipients. Because clinical symptoms and signs of rejection and infection are inadequate and inconsistent, monitoring and diagnosis of rejection rely on both clinical judgment and histological findings. Although histopathological criteria still have some limitations due to the patchy distribution of the immunological mucosal lesions and/or the small size of the endoscopy-guided biopsies, they currently represent the gold standard for the diagnosis of the immunological and infectious complications in InMvTx recipients.

In order to improve the diagnostic yield of enteroscopy and to minimize the level of examiner variability, the endoscopic procedures in InMvTx recipients should be performed by very experienced gastroenterologists familiar with endoscopy in patients with intestinal/multivisceral transplantation.

Additionally, the reports of endoscopic procedures done in InMvTx recipients should include easily identifiable features and utilize descriptive terms with a high degree of correlation and reproducibility. Standardized descriptive terminology among endoscopists can minimize the intra- and interexaminer variability, thus increasing the value of enteroscopy as a reliable diagnostic tool in InMvTx recipients.

The sensitivity, specificity, positive or negative predictive value and accuracy of using the most commonly mentioned mucosal endoscopic findings (erythema, edema, erosions, ulcerations, exudates, pseudomembranes, bleeding, friability, granularity) (Table 2C) as predictors of the immunological (ACR) or infectious (CMV enteritis) complications in the intestinal/multivisceral graft have been prospectively studied by Tabasco-Minguillan et al.

The usefulness of a "normal" endoscopy in predicting the absence of significant histopathological findings showed low predictive values. When all the graft regions were considered, a "normal" endoscopy as indicator of the absence of ACR or CMV presented the following values: sensitivity 55%, specificity 67%, positive predictive value 50%; negative predictive value 71%. Slightly higher values were recorded (sensitivity 56%, specificity 83%, positive predictive value 82%, negative predictive value 59%) when a "normal" endoscopy, as predictor of no ACR or no CMV, was found in the ileal segment of the allograft.

Similarly, the sensitivity, specificity, positive and negative predictive value of ulcers as indicators of ACR, CMV, both or neither have been calculated. When all the grafts were considered, sensitivity (51%) and specificity (71%) in diagnosing ACR were relatively low; the positive predicting value (33%) was also low; the negative predictive value (86%) was higher. When the ileum was considered separately, the sensitivity (100%) and negative predictive value (100%) improved, but specificity (67%) and positive predictive value (33%) did not.

In summary, in a number of cases of intestinal allograft rejection, CMV enteritis or both, the enteroscopic appearance of the intestinal graft has been reported as normal. Consequently, the presence of normal endoscopic features in the intestinal/multivisceral allograft does not exclude immunological or infectious complications.

Considering all graft regions, ulcers present a low sensitivity and a low predictive value for ACR, as they are also found in CMV enteritis. In this setting (all grafts considered), ulcerations are not specific and have a poor positive predictive value in diagnosing rejection. Ulcers in the ileum show improved sensitivity and negative predictive value, decreased specificity and low positive predictive value.

In conclusion, for the time being, enteroscopic examination of the intestinal/multivisceral allograft still presents some methodological limitations: consequently, in InMvTx recipients, endoscopy should not be used as the unique monitoring and diagnostic tool for immunological and/or infectious complications, but it must always be combined with histopathological evaluation, as well as correlated with clinical judgment and "imaging" examinations.

Suggested reading

Abu-Elmagd K, Reyes J, Todo S, Rao A, Lee R, Irish W, Furukawa H, Bueno J, McMichal J, Fawzy AT, Murase N, Demetris J, Rakela J, Fung JJ, Starzl TE (1998) Clinical intestinal transplantation: new perspectives and immunological consideration. J Amer Coll Surg (in press)

Hassanein T, Schade RR, Soldevilla-Pico C, Tabasco-Minguillan J, Abu-Elmagd K, Furukawa H, Kadry Z, Demetris A, Tzakis A, Todo S (1994) Endoscopy is essential for early detection of rejection in small bowel transplant recipients. Transplant Proc 26:1414-1415

Hassanein T, Schade RR, Soldevilla-Pico C, et al (1994) Clinical and endoscopic features of rejection in small bowel transplant recipients. Transplant Proc 26: 1413-1413

Scotti-Foglieni CL, Marino IR, Cillo U, Furukawa H, Abu-Elmagd K, Todo S, Tzakis AG, Fung JJ, Starzl TE (1994) Human intestinal-multivisceral transplantation. In: D'Amico DF, Bassi N, Tedeschi U, Cillo U (eds) Liver transplantation. Procedures and management. Masson, Milano Parigi Barcellona, pp 235-254

Tabasco-Minguillan J, Hutson W, Weber K, Lee RG, Demetris A, Furukawa H, Abu-Elmagd K, Todo S, Rakela J (1996) Prospective evaluation of endoscopy in acute cellular rejection and cytomegalovirus infection. Transplant Proc 28:2778-2779

Tabasco-Minguillan J, Weber K, Nelson F, Hutson W, Furukawa H, Abu-Elmagd K, Todo S, Rakela J (1996) Variability in the interpretations of endoscopic findings in patients with intestinal transplantation. Transplant Proc 28:2775-2776

Uncommon endoscopic appearances of the small bowel mucosa

M. Pennazio, F. P. Rossini

Endoscopic post-surgical surveillance

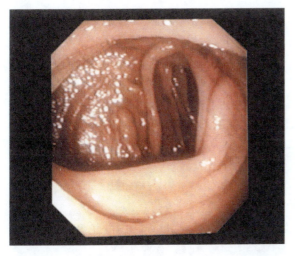

Fig. 1. Normal endoscopic appearance of a termino-terminal jejunal anastomosis in a patient operated on for adenocarcinoma

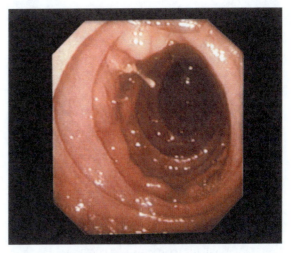

Fig. 2. Termino-terminal jejunal anastomosis in a patient operated on for Crohn's disease. No endoscopic or histological findings of relapse

Uncommon endoscopic appearances of the small bowel mucosa

Giardiasis

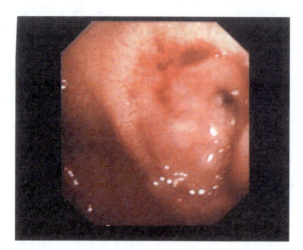

Fig. 3. Stenosis of jejunal anastomosis in a patient operated on for lymphoma

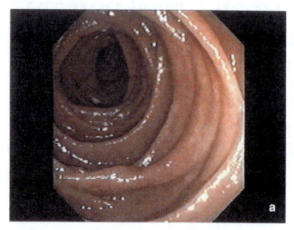

Fig. 5a. *Enteroscopy*: giardiasis. Normal appearance of the mucosa of the jejunum (by courtesy of Dr. P. Meier, Hannover, Germany)

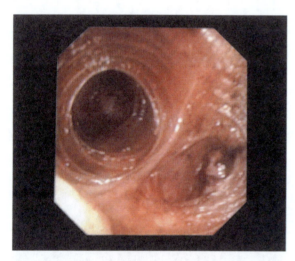

Fig. 4a. Intraoperative enteroscopy. Jejunoileal anastomosis in a patient operated on for Peutz-Jeghers' syndrome. Anastomotic recurrence of a polyp

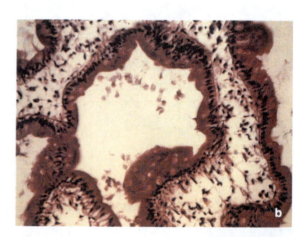

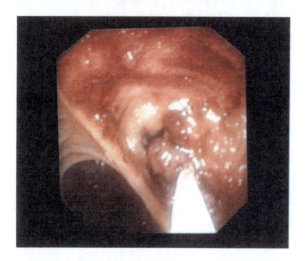

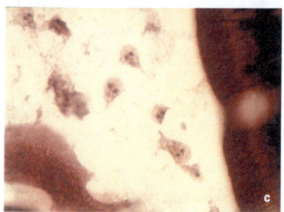

Fig. 5 b,c. *Histology*: numerous trophozoites of *Giardia lamblia* on villous and crypt epithelia (by courtesy of Prof. M. Stolte, Hannover, Germany)

Fig. 4b. Polypectomy

Atlas of Enteroscopy

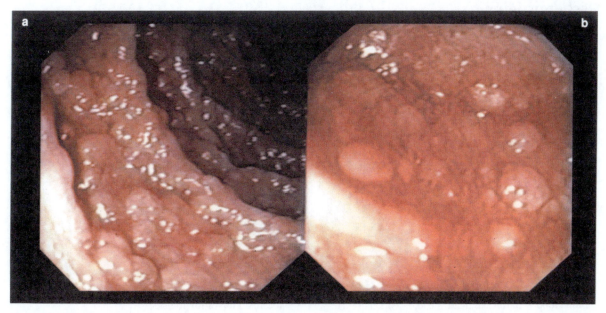

Fig. 6 a,b. Enteroscopy: giardiasis. Multiple small nodules in the jejunal mucosa (by courtesy of Prof. J. Bures, Hradec Kralove, Czech Republic)

Benign lymphoid hyperplasia of the small bowel

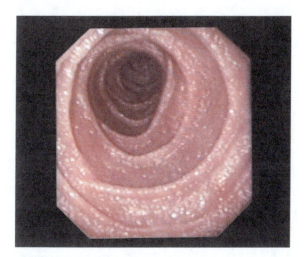

Fig. 7a. Diffuse nodule of the mucosa

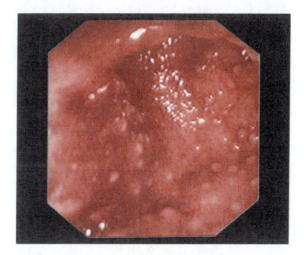

Fig. 7b. Diffuse nodule of the terminal ileum

173

Ischemic jejunitis

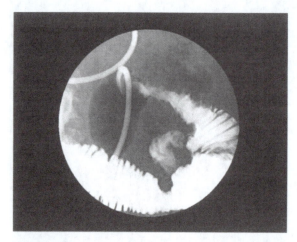

Fig. 8a. *Enteroclysis*: narrowing of the lumen of the first jejunal loop with thickening of the folds, which are irregularly spaced

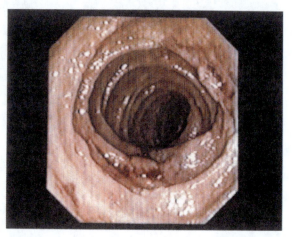

Fig. 8b. *Enteroscopy*: edema of the jejunal mucosa with ulcers on top of the folds

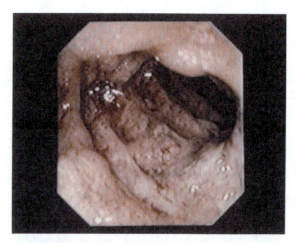

Fig. 8c. *Enteroscopy*: ischemic areas with multiple ulcers. Histology: ischemic jejunitis

Atlas of Enteroscopy

Bleeding lesion in the small bowel

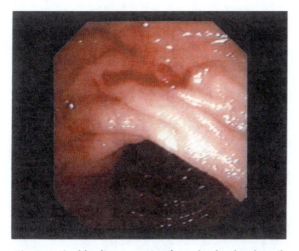

Fig. 9. Active bleeding emerging from the duodenal papilla. This hemorrhage was observed in a patient with chronic pancreatitis and a pancreatitic cyst. Wirsungorrhagia may sometimes be the cause of occult digestive bleeding

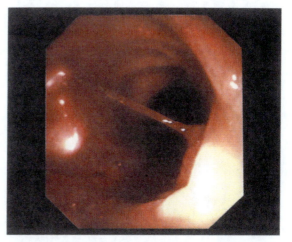

Fig. 10. Active venous bleeding of a jejunal varix that was observed in a cirrhotic patient. Interestingly, no varix was described in the upper gastrointestinal tract. The hemorrhage was controlled after bucrylate injection (by courtesy of Dr. A. Van Gossum, Brussels, Belgium)

Xanthelasma

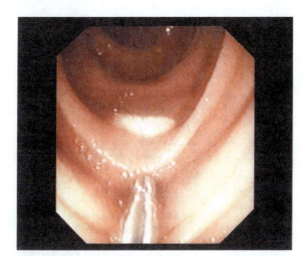

Fig. 11. Jejunal xanthelasma

Printed by Publishers' Graphics LLC